Prostate Cancer Diet Cookbook for Beginners: Recipes and Wisdom for Prostate Health: A Comprehensive 92-Recipe Collection

Kimberly Talbot

Copyright © 2023 Kimberly Talbot

Disclaimer

This book is given for informative purposes only. The information is not meant to be a replacement for professional medical advice, diagnosis, or treatment. Always seek the opinion of your physician or other trained health expert with any inquiries you may have about a medical problem. Never ignore expert medical advice or delay in getting it because of anything you have read in this book.

The author and publisher of this book have tried their best efforts in compiling this content. The author and publisher make no claim or warranties about the correctness, application, suitability, or completeness of the contents. They disclaim all claims (expressed or implied), merchantability, or fitness for any specific purpose. The author and publisher will in no case be held accountable for any loss or other damages, including but not limited to special, incidental, consequential, or other damages. As usual, the assistance of a qualified legal, tax, accounting, or other expert should be obtained.

Any trademarks, service marks, product names, or identified characteristics are presumed to be the property of their respective owners and are used purely for reference. There is no implicit endorsement if we use one of these words.

About the Author

Kimberly Talbot is not only a writer; she's a culinary lover who takes delight in the art of cooking and researching new recipes. Her enthusiasm for the kitchen is not just a creative release but a quest to learn the profound link between food and health.

Married with children, Kimberly's life experiences have molded her outlook on well-being. Witnessing a loved one's fight with prostate cancer kindled a desire inside her to explore the junction of nutrition and prostate health. Her devotion to studying the function of nutrition in encouraging well-being encouraged her to share this information with a larger audience.

In "Prostate cancer diet cookbook for beginners: A Culinary Approach," Kimberly combines her love for writing with her culinary ability to give a guide that goes beyond information—it's a collection of dishes meant to enhance prostate health. Her direct experience has motivated a passion to empower people, families, and caregivers with practical, tasty, and nutritional meal ideas.

Beyond the kitchen, Kimberly is an advocate for holistic well-being. She feels that a balanced and attentive attitude to life is vital to nurturing general wellness. Through her writing, she encourages readers to accompany her on a journey where the pleasure of cooking meets the desire for maximum health.

Kimberly Talbot lives in Charleston, South Carolina, USA, where she continues to experiment with recipes, explore the world of health-conscious food, and find delight in the shared experience of a well-prepared dinner.

Table of content

Introduction

Why Diet Matters for Prostate Health

Welcome to "prostate cancer diet cookbook for beginners." In the pages that follow, we begin on a journey of insight, empowerment, and delectable transformation—a journey that might alter your life or the life of someone you care about.

The journey starts with a simple truth: nutrition has a major impact on our general health, and this is particularly relevant when it comes to prostate health. For males, the prostate is a tiny but crucial organ, responsible for the generation of seminal fluid, and its well-being is inextricably related to our general quality of life.

Prostate cancer is an issue that connects emotionally with people since it's one of the most frequent malignancies afflicting men globally. The good news is that you can make proactive decisions in your everyday life that may minimize your chance of getting prostate cancer and assist in managing the illness if you've already been diagnosed.

This book is your thorough guide to learning how food and nutrition may help your friends in your struggle for prostate health. We'll examine the relevance of a diet rich in key nutrients, foods, and gourmet choices that may make a world of difference.

Throughout these pages, you'll discover practical guidance, delectable recipes, and actionable ideas that appeal to novices. Our objective is to make the transition to a prostate-healthy diet accessible and pleasurable. No previous culinary knowledge is needed; all that's necessary is an open mind, a desire to discover new tastes, and a dedication to your well-being.

We'll dig into the science behind the foods that promote prostate health, explain common myths, and empower you with the knowledge required to make educated dietary choices. Whether you're adopting preventive steps or seeking a route to better manage prostate cancer, you'll find information and inspiration here.

The kitchen is where our trip starts. A well-stocked pantry, smart meal planning, and creative cooking may be the cornerstone of a diet that promotes prostate health. The recipes you'll find on these pages are meant to be both healthful and delightful. From substantial breakfasts to delicious evenings, we've designed a broad selection of cuisine that appeals to your palette and your health.

In addition to recipes, we'll give you example meal plans to ease the process of developing your prostate-healthy diet. We recognize that the road may be tough, but our meal plans can help you get started on the right track.

This book isn't just about eating; it's about adopting a lifestyle that promotes prostate health. We'll cover the value of physical exercise, stress management, and mindful eating. A comprehensive approach is the key to sustaining a healthy and flourishing existence.

Furthermore, the pages ahead will expose you to genuine people who have had their transformational adventures in the domain of prostate health. Their experiences stand as proof of the power of diet and lifestyle in enhancing health and quality of life.

As we continue on this journey together, always remember that information is power, and the decisions you make now may have a tremendous influence on your well-being tomorrow. You're not alone in your attempt; this book is your guide, your partner, and your source of inspiration.

So, let's begin this gastronomic and health journey with an open heart, a questioning mind, and a desire for good change. Together, we'll discover the wonderful and nutritious world of prostate-healthy food, one dish at a time.

Are you ready to adopt a diet that can make a difference in your prostate health and general well-being? Let's get started.

Chapter 1

Understanding Prostate Cancer

What is Prostate Cancer?
In our investigation of prostate health, it's vital to begin with a complete grasp of prostate cancer itself. Prostate cancer, although a name many have heard, frequently stays cloaked in mystery. In this part, we'll throw light on what prostate cancer is, its roots, and the effect it may have on the lives of men.

The Prostate: A Vital Gland

To comprehend prostate cancer, we must first know the importance of the prostate gland in the male body. Nestled under the bladder and around the urethra like a protective donut, the prostate is a tiny, walnut-sized organ. Although it's sometimes disregarded in talks about the male reproductive system, the prostate plays a key function.

The fundamental function of the prostate is to create seminal fluid, a key component of semen. Seminal fluid is not merely a neutral container for sperm but a critical nourishing and transport medium. It includes enzymes, proteins, and nutrients that sustain the sperm on its route to conception. In essence, the prostate gland is a co-pilot in the miracle of human procreation.

The Emergence of Prostate Cancer

Prostate cancer, as the name indicates, is cancer that begins in the prostate. Like other malignancies, it starts with the uncontrolled growth and division of cells. In the case of prostate cancer, this aberrant cell proliferation happens in the prostate gland itself. Over time, these malignant cells might aggregate, producing a lump or tumor.

Not every prostate cancer is the same, and this is a key point of knowledge. Prostate cancer may vary in terms of its aggressiveness and how rapidly it develops. Some people may have what is known as "low-grade" prostate cancer, which tends to be slow-growing and less likely to spread beyond the prostate. On the other hand, "high-grade" prostate cancer is more aggressive and may spread to surrounding tissues or even distant sections of the body.

The course of the illness may be impacted by several variables, including genetics, lifestyle, and treatment decisions. This is why knowing prostate cancer, its risk factors, and early detection procedures is crucial. By diagnosing and managing prostate cancer in its early stages, people have a greater chance of effective treatment and enhanced quality of life.

The Importance of Early Detection

Prostate cancer is frequently labeled a "silent killer" because it may grow without visible signs in its early stages. This is why frequent tests and check-ups are vital, particularly as men get older. The two basic techniques of early detection are the prostate-specific antigen (PSA) blood test and the digital rectal exam (DRE).

The PSA blood test analyzes the amount of prostate-specific antigen in the blood, which may be raised in the presence of prostate cancer. The DRE is a physical examination in which a healthcare clinician analyzes the prostate's size, shape, and texture via the rectum.

It's crucial to highlight that a high PSA level or an abnormal DRE test doesn't inevitably indicate prostate cancer. Further testing, such as a prostate biopsy, may be indicated to confirm the diagnosis. These exams, although vital, may be scary and distressing for many men. However, the potential advantages of early diagnosis and treatment greatly exceed the pain of the diagnostic procedure. Knowledge is your ally in the quest to preserve prostate health. Understanding what prostate cancer is and how it might develop is the first step toward empowerment.

Risk Factors and Early Detection

Prostate cancer, like any other illness, doesn't discriminate. It may afflict guys of various backgrounds and areas of life. However, some variables may raise the chance of getting prostate cancer, and early identification plays a vital role in treating this health concern.

Age: The Most Significant Risk Factor

Age is likely the most important risk factor for prostate cancer. This is an irrefutable reality, and although it can be difficult to recognize, it's vital. Prostate cancer is infrequent in males under the age of 40. However, as men get older, the probability of having prostate cancer greatly rises.

It's typically suggested that men start considering prostate cancer screening with their healthcare professionals at approximately age 50, or even earlier if there are other risk factors present. Regular tests are vital to discover the illness in its early stages when it's more controllable and curable.

Family History: A Crucial Piece of the Puzzle

Family history is another key component in the arena of prostate cancer. If you have a father, brother, or any close male relatives who've been diagnosed with prostate cancer, your risk is raised. The danger is much larger if numerous family members have been afflicted.

Genetics may play a role in these family clusters of prostate cancer. Therefore, if you have a family history of the condition, you should be extremely careful about your prostate health. This doesn't imply that you're destined to acquire prostate cancer, but it highlights the need for early identification and proactive health management.

Race and Ethnicity: Disparities in Risk

Prostate cancer doesn't impact all guys equally. There are considerable racial and ethnic inequalities in prostate cancer risk. Among these differences, African American males have a greater risk compared to other racial and ethnic groups. They are not only more likely to be diagnosed with prostate cancer but also more likely to develop severe forms of the illness.

In contrast, Asian and Hispanic men appear to have a decreased chance of acquiring prostate cancer. The causes for these discrepancies are complicated and currently being investigated. Genetics, access to healthcare, and environmental factors may all influence.

Diet and Lifestyle: A Controllable Risk Factor

While age, family history, and race are characteristics you can't control, your food and lifestyle are areas where you have a say in minimizing your risk of prostate cancer. Studies have revealed that various food and lifestyle choices might impact your risk. Here are some crucial aspects to consider:

- Diet: A diet heavy in red and processed meats and low in fruits and vegetables has been connected with an elevated risk of prostate cancer. Conversely, a diet rich in plant-based foods, antioxidants, and certain minerals may be protective.

- Physical exercise: Engaging in regular physical exercise has been associated with a decreased chance of acquiring prostate cancer. Exercise may help control weight and lower the risk of chronic illnesses, which may add to prostate cancer risk.

- Obesity: Maintaining a healthy weight is vital for prostate health. Obesity is connected with an increased risk of aggressive prostate cancer and a greater chance of recurrence following therapy.

- Smoking: Smoking is not only a substantial risk factor for different malignancies but may also be related to an elevated chance of aggressive prostate cancer.

Environmental Factors: A Potential Influence

Some environmental elements are being researched for their potential relation to prostate cancer. Exposure to specific chemicals or poisons, such as Agent Orange or cadmium, is being researched for possible ties to prostate cancer risk. However, the evidence in this area is not yet conclusive.

The Role of Early Detection

While identifying the risk factors is critical, early diagnosis is crucial. Detecting prostate cancer in its early stages considerably enhances the odds of effective therapy. Routine check-ups and screenings allow for the detection of possible problems before symptoms appear.

The two basic techniques of early detection are the PSA blood test and the digital rectal exam (DRE). The PSA test analyzes the amount of prostate-specific antigen in the blood, which may be raised in the presence of prostate cancer. The DRE is a physical examination in which a healthcare clinician analyzes the prostate's size, shape, and texture via the rectum.

It's crucial to recognize that an increased PSA level or an abnormal DRE test doesn't inevitably indicate prostate cancer. Further testing, such as a prostate biopsy, may be indicated to confirm the diagnosis.

As we continue ahead in our quest toward prostate health, this information is your armor, and early diagnosis is your shield. By recognizing the risk factors, you may make educated choices about your health and take proactive efforts to lower your risk. Regular tests may spot possible concerns before they become overwhelming obstacles.

Our journey to study prostate health via food choices and lifestyle starts with a thorough awareness of the terrain. Armed with this information, you'll be better positioned to make educated choices about your health and lower your chance of prostate cancer. The trip continues, and we're ready to take the next step.

The Connection Between Diet and Prostate Cancer

The relationship between nutrition and prostate cancer is a topic of considerable interest in medical study. While numerous variables contribute to prostate cancer risk, the foods we consume may play a major influence. In this part, we'll look into the relationship between nutrition and prostate cancer, studying the influence of dietary choices on your prostate health.

A Balancing Act: The Power of Nutrition

Our bodies need a careful balance of nutrients to operate efficiently. When this equilibrium is broken, it may lead to health complications, including an increased risk of cancer. In the context of prostate health, various nutrients, and dietary ingredients have been related to either a greater or decreased risk of prostate cancer.

Antioxidants: These molecules, present in numerous fruits and vegetables, play a critical function in neutralizing damaging free radicals in the body. Free radicals may harm cells and DNA, possibly leading to cancer formation. Antioxidant-rich foods may help protect the prostate and minimize the chance of cancer.

Cruciferous Vegetables: Vegetables including broccoli, cauliflower, and Brussels sprouts have bioactive chemicals that may have preventive benefits against prostate cancer. These substances are considered to help inhibit the formation of cancer cells.

Lycopene: Lycopene is a potent antioxidant present in tomatoes and tomato-based products. Research has revealed that a diet high in lycopene may be connected with a decreased risk of prostate cancer.

Selenium: Selenium is a trace element present in nuts, seeds, and some cereals. Adequate selenium consumption may be connected to a lower risk of prostate cancer.

Fiber: A diet rich in fiber, particularly from whole grains and fruits, helps improve digestive health and may lead to a lower risk of prostate cancer.

Good Fats: While saturated and trans fats found in red and processed meats are associated with an increased risk of prostate cancer, good fats, such as those in nuts, seeds, and fatty fish, may have preventive benefits.

Processed Meats: On the other side, diets heavy in processed meats like bacon, sausages, and hot dogs have been connected with an increased risk of prostate cancer. These meats typically include preservatives and chemicals that may lead to cancer development.

Dietary Patterns: The general pattern of your diet counts as well. A Mediterranean-style diet, typified by a high consumption of fruits, vegetables, whole grains, and healthy fats, has been connected with a lower risk of prostate cancer. On the other hand, a Western-style diet, which is strong in red meat, processed foods, and sweets, may enhance the risk.

Weight Management: Maintaining a healthy weight is crucial for prostate health. Obesity has been associated with an increased risk of aggressive prostate cancer and a greater chance of recurrence following therapy.

Alcohol Consumption: Excessive alcohol consumption has been connected with an increased risk of prostate cancer. Limiting alcohol intake is a sensible decision for both prostate health and general well-being.

It's vital to recognize that although these dietary factors may have a role in prostate cancer risk, they're not the primary drivers. A mix of variables, including genetics, age, and environmental effects, adds to an individual's risk.

As we advance on our path toward a prostate-healthy diet, you'll find practical solutions, tasty recipes, and meal plans that combine these cancer-fighting ingredients. A thoughtful approach to your food choices may have a substantial influence on your prostate health.

Knowledge is your ally, and the understanding of the relationship between food and prostate cancer is your compass.

We're on the way to learning how food may be a vital factor in your journey to prostate health. As we examine the power of nutrition and its capacity to minimize risk, support treatment, and increase quality of life, we'll provide you with the skills you need to make educated decisions for your well-being.

Chapter 2

The Prostate-Healthy Diet Basics

The Power of Whole Foods
Now that we've established a solid knowledge of prostate cancer and the function of nutrition in prostate health, it's time to dig deeper into the core of our adventure. In this chapter, we'll examine the basic concepts of a prostate-healthy diet, starting with the tremendous power of whole foods.

Whole Foods: Nature's Gift to Your Prostate

Whole foods are the hidden heroes of a balanced and healthy diet. They are foods in their most natural, unadulterated state—items that are as near to their original form as possible. Whole foods contain a broad selection of possibilities, including fruits, vegetables, whole grains, legumes, nuts, seeds, and lean meats.

Why are whole foods so crucial in the context of prostate health? The solution lies in their purity and nutritional density. These foods contain a treasure trove of vitamins, minerals, fiber, antioxidants, and phytochemicals that act in harmony to protect and promote the prostate.

Nutrient Density: Whole foods are loaded with important nutrients. They contain a rich amount of vitamins and minerals, such as vitamins A, C, and E, and the mineral selenium, all of which have been connected with prostate health. Nutrient-dense meals feed your body with the building blocks it needs to perform efficiently.

Fiber: Whole foods are a key source of dietary fiber. A high-fiber diet, largely from fruits, vegetables, and whole grains, may improve your digestive system and help maintain a healthy weight. Fiber may also contribute to a lower risk of prostate cancer.

Antioxidants: The antioxidant content of whole foods is a robust defense against oxidative stress. Free radicals, which may harm cells and DNA, are neutralized by antioxidants. Fruits and vegetables are especially rich in antioxidants, offering a crucial defense for your prostate.

Phytochemicals: Whole foods include diverse phytochemicals, and plant substances that provide distinct health advantages. For prostate health, foods like tomatoes (rich in lycopene), cruciferous vegetables (containing sulforaphane), and green tea (abundant in catechins) are recognized for their prostate-protective phytochemicals.

Balanced Nutrition: Whole foods give a balanced nutritional profile. They supply an assortment of macronutrients (carbohydrates, proteins, and healthy fats) and micronutrients (vitamins and minerals) that your body needs to operate harmoniously. This balance is critical for general health and especially for prostate health.

Full and fulfilling: Whole meals are often more full and fulfilling than processed alternatives. This satiety may help you maintain a healthy weight, a vital component of prostate health.

Digestive Health: The fiber in whole meals helps digestive health and regularity. A healthy digestive system is vital for the disposal of waste and pollutants, minimizing the stress on your body.

Inflammation Management: Whole foods have anti-inflammatory effects. Chronic inflammation is thought to be a contributing cause of several illnesses, including cancer. A diet rich in anti-inflammatory foods may help regulate inflammation and support your body's natural defenses.

Incorporating whole foods into your diet is a cornerstone of prostate health. While these meals provide enormous advantages, they also have the advantage of being tasty and diverse. The colors, tastes, and textures contained in whole foods may add brightness to your meals, making the road to a prostate-healthy diet not just beneficial but delightful.

The beauty of whole foods is that they're accessible and adaptable to a range of culinary tastes. Whether you're a lover of fresh salads, substantial stews, or vivid smoothies, there's a place for whole foods in your nutritional repertoire.

Key Nutrients for Prostate Health

As we go further into the core of a prostate-healthy diet, it's critical to identify and understand the main nutrients that play a significant role in supporting your prostate. These nutrients are the building blocks of your diet, and they're vital for preserving prostate health and minimizing the chance of prostate cancer.

Let's discover the nutrients that your prostate will thank you for.

Vitamin A: Vitamin A is a potent antioxidant that strengthens the immune system and helps protect the prostate from oxidative stress. It's often found in orange and yellow fruits and vegetables, such as carrots and sweet potatoes, as well as in leafy greens and dairy products.

Vitamin C: Another strong antioxidant, vitamin C, plays a critical function in prostate health by neutralizing free radicals and strengthening the immune system. Citrus fruits, strawberries, and bell peppers are good sources of vitamin C.

Vitamin E: Vitamin E is yet another antioxidant that may help protect the prostate from damage caused by free radicals. Nuts, seeds, and vegetable oils, notably sunflower and safflower oil, are important sources of vitamin E.

Selenium: Selenium is a trace element that has been related to a lower risk of prostate cancer. It functions as an antioxidant and is present in foods including Brazil nuts, seafood, chicken, and whole grains.

Lycopene: Lycopene is a carotenoid antioxidant found in red and pink fruits and vegetables, with tomatoes being the most well-known source. Lycopene has been connected with a decreased incidence of prostate cancer and is a cornerstone in a prostate-healthy diet.

Zinc: Zinc is a vital element for prostate health. It's engaged in several physiological functions and promotes a healthy immune system. Zinc-rich foods include oysters, lean meats, and dairy products.

Fiber: Dietary fiber, mostly found in fruits, vegetables, and whole grains, is necessary for digestive health. It helps maintain regular bowel motions and correlates to a lower risk of prostate cancer.

Omega-3 Fatty Acids: These healthful fats, found in fatty fish like salmon and trout, flaxseeds, and walnuts, have anti-inflammatory qualities. They may help decrease inflammation in the prostate and contribute to overall wellness.

Phytochemicals: Phytochemicals are bioactive molecules found in plants that provide distinct health advantages. Some of the most well-known phytochemicals for prostate health are sulforaphane (found in cruciferous foods like broccoli), catechins (rich in green tea), and curcumin (found in turmeric).

Folate (Vitamin B9): Folate is a B vitamin that assists DNA repair and synthesis. It's usually found in leafy green vegetables, legumes, and fortified cereals.

Fiber: Dietary fiber is a dietary superstar, boosting digestive health and contributing to general well-being. It's bountiful in fruits, vegetables, whole grains, and legumes.

Water: While not a nutrient per se, proper hydration is crucial for prostate health. Staying well-hydrated promotes your body's natural detoxification processes and helps preserve overall health.

Each of these nutrients performs a particular purpose in supporting your prostate and overall well-being. By integrating a range of foods high in these critical nutrients into your diet, you'll be taking big strides toward a prostate-healthy eating plan. The recipes and meal plans in this trip are intended to contain these prostate-protective nutrients, making it simple and enjoyable to feed your prostate.

Foods to Embrace and Avoid

In our path to improved prostate health via diet, it's not just about the nutrients and healthy foods we welcome into our lives but also about being aware of the choices we make. Some meals have been connected with prostate health advantages, while others may raise the risk of prostate cancer. Here, we'll examine the meals to embrace and those to avoid.

Foods to Embrace: Prostate-Protective Choices

- Tomatoes: Tomatoes are recognized for their lycopene content, a potent antioxidant linked with a decreased risk of prostate cancer. Include fresh tomatoes, tomato sauce, and tomato-based meals in your diet.

- Cruciferous Vegetables: Broccoli, cauliflower, Brussels sprouts, and kale are high in sulforaphane, a chemical that may have preventative benefits against prostate cancer. Enjoy these vegetables in salads, stir-fries, or steamed as side dishes.

- Berries: Berries like strawberries, blueberries, and raspberries are not only tasty but also full of antioxidants and phytochemicals that support prostate health. Add them to your breakfast or munch on them during the day.

- Fatty Fish: Salmon, trout, mackerel, and sardines are rich in omega-3 fatty acids, which have anti-inflammatory qualities. Incorporate these fish into your diet frequently.

- Nuts and Seeds: Almonds, walnuts, flaxseeds, and chia seeds are wonderful providers of healthy fats, fiber, and critical nutrients. Snack on them, sprinkle them over yogurt or use them as toppings in your meals.

- Green Tea: Green tea includes catechins, which have been connected with many health benefits, including possible prostate cancer prevention. Enjoy a cup of green tea as part of your daily routine.

- Leafy Greens: Spinach, kale, and other leafy greens are rich in nutrients, including folate, which promotes prostate health. Incorporate them into salads, smoothies, or side dishes.

- Pomegranate: Pomegranate is a fruit-laden with antioxidants and has been connected to possible prostate cancer protection. You may take pomegranate juice or fresh pomegranate seeds.

- Olive Oil: Extra virgin olive oil is a source of healthful monounsaturated fats. Use it for salad dressings and in cooking to get its possible health advantages.

- Legumes: Beans, lentils, and chickpeas are good sources of fiber and plant-based protein. They may be the foundation for soups, stews, and plant-based cuisines.

Foods to Avoid or Limit: Potential Prostate Health Risks

- Red and Processed Meats: High intake of red meats (beef, lamb, and hog) and processed meats (such as bacon, sausages, and hot dogs) has been connected with an elevated risk of prostate cancer. Limit your consumption of these meats.

- Sugary Foods and Beverages: A diet heavy in sugary foods and beverages may lead to weight gain and obesity, which is related to an elevated risk of aggressive prostate cancer. Reduce your intake of sugary goods.

- High-Dairy Diets: Some studies show that a high diet of dairy products, especially high-fat dairy, may enhance the risk of prostate cancer. Consider minimizing full-fat dairy and exploring dairy substitutes.

- Trans Fats: Trans fats are present in several processed and fried meals and have been related to an elevated risk of aggressive prostate cancer. Check food labels and avoid goods containing trans fats.

- Excessive Alcohol: Excessive alcohol drinking has been related to an increased risk of prostate cancer. If you drink alcohol, do so in moderation.

- Salt: Diets heavy in salt, generally coming from processed and fast meals, may be associated with an elevated risk of prostate cancer. Opt for low-sodium choices wherever feasible.

Remember, making great eating choices is not about deprivation but about balance and attentiveness. By embracing prostate-protective foods and being conscious of those that may represent a danger, you may take big strides toward prostate health.

Chapter 3

Setting Up Your Kitchen for Success

Stocking a Prostate-Healthy Pantry
A well-stocked kitchen is the backbone of a successful path toward a prostate-healthy diet. It's your refuge, your studio, and your culinary canvas, where you'll create delicious and healthful meals. In this chapter, we'll instruct you on how to set up your kitchen for success, beginning with the critical step of filling a prostate-healthy pantry. A well-equipped pantry sets the basis for healthful cuisine. Here's a list of crucial goods to have in your prostate-healthy pantry:

- Whole Grains: Whole grains including brown rice, quinoa, whole wheat pasta, and oats are good providers of fiber and minerals. They serve as a basis for many healthful meals.

- Canned Tomatoes: Canned tomatoes, whether whole, chopped, or crushed, are versatile foods high in lycopene. They constitute the foundation for many sauces, soups, and stews.

- Low-Sodium Broth: Vegetable, chicken, or beef broth is a vital addition to your cupboard for seasoning soups, sauces, and cereals. Opt for low-sodium variants to limit salt consumption.

- Canned Beans: Stock up on canned beans including black beans, kidney beans, and chickpeas. They're a simple source of plant-based protein and fiber for salads, stews, and more.

- Canned Tuna or Salmon: Canned fish is a fast and protein-rich choice for salads and sandwiches. Look for water-packed choices to minimize additional fats.

- Nuts and Seeds: Store a variety of nuts and seeds, such as almonds, walnuts, flaxseeds, and chia seeds. They offer crispness and nutrition to your meals and snacks.

- Olive Oil: Extra virgin olive oil is a heart-healthy fat and a tasty addition to your cupboard for sautéing, sauces, and roasting.

- Whole Wheat Flour: If you like baking, choose whole wheat flour as a more healthy alternative for bread, muffins, and other sweets.

- Dried Herbs and Spices: A well-stocked spice rack is your secret weapon for adding flavor without additional salt or fat. Include essentials like garlic powder, oregano, basil, and others.

- Vinegar: Balsamic, red wine, and apple cider vinegar are diverse alternatives for dressings and marinades.

- Whole Grain Pasta: Choose whole wheat or legume-based pasta for increased fiber and nutrients in your pasta meals.

- Natural Sweeteners: Opt for natural sweeteners like honey or maple syrup as alternatives to refined sugar for occasional sweetening.

- Canned Fruits: Keep canned fruits like peaches, pears, or pineapple in natural juices for a fast and healthful dessert alternative.

- Nut Butter: Peanut, almond, or other nut butter may be a delightful and protein-rich addition to your cupboard.

- Whole Grain Cereals: Stock whole grain cereals, such as oats or whole grain bran, for a fiber-rich morning choice.

- Dried Fruits: Dried fruits like apricots, raisins, or cranberries may be a healthful addition to cereals and salads.

- Whole Grain Crackers: These are excellent for a healthful snack or a basis for appetizers with hummus or nut butter.

- Herbal Teas: Herbal teas are a calming and caffeine-free alternative for drinks.

- Low-Sodium Soy Sauce: This is a taste enhancer for many Asian-inspired foods. Opt for the low-sodium option to manage salt consumption.

- Canned veggies: While fresh is ideal, canned veggies like peas, maize, or green beans may be beneficial in a crisis.

By having these things in your cupboard, you'll be well-prepared to whip up prostate-healthy meals whenever the inspiration hits. A well-organized pantry not only simplifies meal preparation but also encourages you to make healthier choices. Your path to prostate health begins right here, with every item you keep, and every meal you construct.

Essential Kitchen Tools

A well-stocked kitchen is not complete without the necessary equipment to help you prepare and cook your prostate-healthy meals. Here's a list of necessary kitchen items that will make your culinary adventure more efficient and enjoyable:

- Cutting Board: Invest in a good-quality cutting board made of wood or plastic. It should be big enough to comfortably chop and prepare food.

- Chef's Knife: A sharp chef's knife is your culinary workhorse. It's multifunctional and important for chopping, dicing, and slicing.

- Paring Knife: A tiny paring knife is great for precise chores like peeling, trimming, and other delicate cutting.

- Vegetable Peeler: An excellent vegetable peeler makes rapid work of peeling fruits and vegetables.

- Measuring Cups and Spoons: Accurate measures are vital for cooking. A set of measuring cups and spoons is a must-have.

- Mixing Bowls: A selection of mixing bowls in various sizes is convenient for combining, tossing, and marinating items.

- Saucepan: A saucepan with a cover is necessary for cooking sauces, soups, and cereals.

- Frying Pan: A decent non-stick frying pan is adaptable for sautéing and frying without unnecessary oil.

- Stockpot: A big stockpot is useful for preparing soups, stews, and simmering large amounts of grains or noodles.

- Baking Sheets: Baking sheets are helpful for roasting veggies, preparing sheet pan dinners, and baking.

- Strainer/Colander: A strainer or colander is useful for draining pasta, cleaning vegetables, and sifting.

- Blender or Food Processor: A blender or food processor may be used to prepare smoothies, soups, sauces, and even homemade nut butter.

- Salad Spinner: A salad spinner makes washing and drying lush greens a snap.

- Grater/Zester: A grater is helpful for shredding cheese and vegetables, while a zester is fantastic for adding citrus zest to meals.

- Can Opener: A dependable can opener is crucial for accessing canned products in your pantry.

- Tongs: Tongs are multifunctional for flipping, tossing, and dishing.

- Whisk: A whisk is great for combining and emulsifying dressings, sauces, and batters.

- Microwave-Safe Containers: Microwave-safe containers are handy for reheating leftovers.

- Oven Mitts: Protect your hands when handling hot cookware with oven mitts.

- Timer: A timer will help you keep track of cooking times and avoid overcooking.

- Cutting Board Mats: Cutting board mats are a hygienic and space-saving method to prep materials.

- Digital Thermometer: A digital thermometer guarantees your meats and dishes are cooked to the appropriate temperature.

- Kitchen Scale: A kitchen scale is helpful for accurate measures, particularly for baking.

- Canisters and Storage Container: Keep your pantry organized using canisters and storage containers to store dry foods and pantry staples.

- Ladle: A ladle is useful for serving soups and stews.

Having these basic kitchen items on hand can speed up your cooking process and make it simpler to produce tasty and prostate-healthy meals.

Smart Shopping Tips

The basis of a prostate-healthy diet starts at the grocery store. Here are some smart shopping suggestions to help you make wholesome and educated decisions while you stock up on groceries for your meals:

- Plan Your Meals: Before going to the shop, plan your meals for the week. Create a list of the things you'll need, then stick to it. Planning helps you avoid impulsive purchases.

- Shop the Perimeter: The perimeter of the grocery store often stores fresh vegetables, lean proteins, and dairy items. Focus on these areas for healthier choices.

- Read Labels: Take the time to read food labels. Look for items with shorter ingredient lists and minimum added sugars, bad fats, and salt.

- Choose entire Foods: Opt for entire, unprocessed foods wherever feasible. Fresh fruits and vegetables, whole grains, and lean proteins should form the base of your shopping.

- Limit Processed Foods: Processed foods frequently include high quantities of salt, harmful fats, and additives. Limit your purchases of these things.

- Compare Prices: Compare prices and sizes to discover the greatest deal. Often, purchasing in bulk or picking store-brand items might save you money.

- Buy Seasonal Produce: Seasonal fruits and vegetables are generally fresher and more cheap. They're also better for the environment.

- Choose Lean Proteins: Select lean cuts of meat, poultry, and fish to limit saturated fat consumption. You may also investigate plant-based protein sources like beans and tofu.

- Check for Sales and Coupons: Be on the lookout for specials, discounts, and coupons to save money on your groceries.

- Frozen and Canned Options: Don't neglect frozen and canned fruits and vegetables. They may be just as healthy as fresh and have a longer shelf life.

- Avoid impulsive Buys: Stick to your list and avoid impulsive purchases that might be heavy in sugar, harmful fats, or empty calories.

- Shop When Not Hungry: Avoid grocery shopping when you're hungry since you're more inclined to make less nutritious selections.

- Limit Sugary and Processed Snacks: Minimize your purchase of sugary snacks, cookies, and chips. Instead, choose for healthy snack alternatives like almonds, yogurt, and fresh fruit.

- Read Nutrition Facts: Pay attention to the nutrition data on packaged items. Look for reduced salt, sugar, and saturated fat levels.

- Stock Up on Pantry Essentials: Always keep key pantry staples, such as whole grains, canned tomatoes, beans, and olive oil, easily accessible.

- Stick to the outside Aisles: Grocery shops generally display healthier, fresh products around the outside aisles. These sectors include the vegetable, meat, and dairy divisions.

- Bring Your Reusable Bags: Reducing plastic waste is ecologically beneficial. Bringing your reusable shopping bags is an easy way to help sustainability.

By following these smart purchasing strategies, you'll not only load your cart with prostate-healthy products but also make your excursions to the grocery store more efficient and budget-friendly. Your buying decisions are a key part of your road to a prostate-healthy diet, and they set the tone for your culinary adventures in the kitchen. Each decision you make at the shop is a step toward a better, more nutritious lifestyle.

Chapter 4

Breakfasts to Start Your Day Right

Energizing Breakfast Recipes
Breakfast is the cornerstone of your day, and it's the ideal time to nourish your body with energetic, prostate-healthy foods. In this part, we'll examine some tasty and wholesome breakfast dishes meant to begin your morning and give you the energy you need to conquer the day.

Prostate-Boosting Smoothie Bowl

This vivid and satisfying smoothie bowl is filled with ingredients that promote prostate health. The mix of bright berries, nuts, seeds, and nutritious grains will keep you energetic throughout the morning.

Ingredients

- 1/2 cup mixed berries (strawberries, blueberries, raspberries)
- 1 small banana
- 1/4 cup rolled oats
- 1 tablespoon flaxseeds
- 1 tablespoon chia seeds
- 1/2 cup low-fat Greek yogurt
- 1/4 cup almond milk (or your choice of milk)
- 1 tablespoon honey or maple syrup (optional, for sweetness)
- Toppings: sliced almonds, more berries, and a sprinkle of granola

Instructions

- In a blender, combine the mixed berries, bananas, rolled oats, flaxseeds, chia seeds, Greek yogurt, and almond milk.

- Blend until you obtain a smooth and creamy consistency. If you like a sweeter flavor, you may add honey or maple syrup at this point.

- Pour the smoothie mixture into a bowl.

- Top with sliced almonds, additional berries, and a sprinkling of granola for more texture and taste.

- Enjoy your prostate-boosting smoothie bowl as a bright and healthy way to start your day.

Avocado and Egg Breakfast Toast

This tasty morning bread is rich in heart-healthy fats and protein. Avocado and eggs are a power combo that gives lasting energy, and the whole-grain bread adds fiber to keep you satisfied.

Ingredients

- 1 slice of whole grain bread (or your choice of bread)
- 1/2 ripe avocado
- 1 poached or fried egg
- Salt and pepper to taste
- A sprinkle of red pepper flakes (optional, for a kick)
- Fresh herbs (such as chives or cilantro) for garnish

Instructions

- Toast your piece of whole-grain bread until it achieves your chosen degree of crispiness.

- While the bread is browning, split the ripe avocado in half, remove the pit, and scoop out the meat. Mash it with a fork and add a touch of salt and pepper. You may also add red pepper flakes for a little spiciness.

- Poach or fry one egg to your taste, keeping the yolk slightly runny for a creamy texture.

- Spread the mashed avocado over the toasted bread.

- Gently lay the poached or cooked egg on top of the avocado spread.

- Garnish with fresh herbs, a touch extra salt and pepper, and more red pepper flakes if preferred.

- Your avocado and egg breakfast toast is ready to offer you a delightful and nutrient-rich start to your day.

Greek Yogurt Parfait with Berries and Nuts

This Greek yogurt parfait is a delicious combination of creamy yogurt, sweet berries, and crunchy almonds. It's a protein-packed breakfast that's both filling and invigorating.

Ingredients

- 1 cup Greek yogurt (low-fat or non-fat)
- 1/2 cup mixed berries (strawberries, blueberries, raspberries)
- 2 tablespoons chopped nuts (such as almonds or walnuts)
- 1 tablespoon honey or maple syrup (optional, for sweetness)
- 1/4 teaspoon cinnamon (optional, for flavor)
- Fresh mint leaves for garnish

Instructions

- In a glass or dish, layer half of the Greek yogurt.

- Add a layer of mixed berries on top of the yogurt.

- Sprinkle chopped nuts over the fruit.

- Drizzle honey or maple syrup over the nuts for extra sweetness, if preferred. You may also add a pinch of cinnamon for added taste.

- Layer the leftover Greek yogurt on top of the nuts.

- Garnish with fresh mint leaves for a punch of freshness.

- Your Greek yogurt parfait is ready to give you with a protein-rich and refreshing morning meal.

Spinach and Mushroom Omelette

This substantial omelette is a flavorful pleasure that's full of protein, vitamins, and minerals. The mix of spinach and mushrooms blasts flavor and nourishment to your morning.

Ingredients

- 2 large eggs
- 1/2 cup fresh spinach leaves
- 1/4 cup sliced mushrooms
- 2 tablespoons diced onion
- 1 tablespoon olive oil
- Salt and pepper to taste
- 2 tablespoons shredded low-fat cheese (optional)

Instructions

- Heat the olive oil in a non-stick pan over medium heat.

- Add the chopped onion and sliced mushrooms to the pan. Sauté until the mushrooms are soft and the onions are transparent.

- Add the fresh spinach leaves to the pan and simmer until wilted.

- In a separate dish, beat the eggs and season with a touch of salt and pepper.

- Pour the beaten eggs over the sautéed veggies in the pan.

- Cook the omelette until the sides are firm, and the middle is slightly runny.

- If preferred, sprinkle low-fat cheese over one-half of the omelet.

- Carefully fold the omelet in half to cover the cheese, making a half-moon shape.

- Cook for another minute or until the cheese has melted.

- Slide the omelet onto a dish, chop in two, and serve.

Chia Seed Pudding with Fresh Fruit

Chia seeds are small nutritional powerhouses filled with fiber, protein, and healthy fats. When wet, they morph into a pudding-like consistency that's excellent for a tasty and energy-boosting breakfast.

Ingredients

- 3 tablespoons chia seeds
- 1 cup almond milk (or your choice of milk)
- 1/2 teaspoon vanilla extract

- 1 tablespoon honey or maple syrup (optional, for sweetness)
- Fresh fruit for topping (e.g., sliced strawberries, kiwi, and blueberries)

Instructions

- In a dish, blend the chia seeds, almond milk, and vanilla essence.

- If you like sweetness, add honey or maple syrup at this point. Mix thoroughly. ·

- Cover the bowl and refrigerate the chia seed mixture for at least 4 hours or overnight. The chia seeds will absorb the liquid and form a pudding-like consistency.

- When ready to serve, pour the chia seed pudding into a dish or glass.

- Top with fresh fruit, such as sliced strawberries, kiwi, and blueberries.

- Your chia seed pudding with fresh fruit is ready to offer you a fiber-rich and nutrient-packed morning.

Whole Grain Pancakes with Fruit Topping

Indulge in the fluffy bliss of whole-grain pancakes topped with a burst of fresh fruit. These pancakes give a delicious start to your day, and their nutritious grains provide enduring energy.

Ingredients

- 1 cup whole wheat flour
- 1 tablespoon honey or maple syrup
- 1 teaspoon baking powder
- 1/4 teaspoon salt
- 1 cup almond milk (or your choice of milk)
- 1 large egg
- 1/2 teaspoon vanilla extract
- Sliced fresh fruit (e.g., banana, strawberries, or blueberries) for topping

- Maple syrup or yogurt (optional, for extra flavor)

Instructions

- In a bowl, mix the whole wheat flour, honey or maple syrup, baking powder, and salt.

- In a separate dish, whisk the egg and add the almond milk and vanilla essence.

- Combine the wet ingredients with the dry components and mix until the batter is smooth.

- Heat a non-stick skillet or griddle over medium-high heat.

- Pour 1/4 cup of the pancake batter onto the heated skillet for each pancake.

- Cook until you see bubbles on the top, then turn and cook the other side until golden brown.

- Serve the whole grain pancakes with sliced fresh fruit on top.

- If preferred, sprinkle with maple syrup or add a dollop of yogurt for added taste.

Oatmeal with Berries and Almonds

Oatmeal is a traditional breakfast option that's robust, nourishing, and full of fiber. Adding fresh berries and almonds boosts both taste and nutrients, making it a go-to breakfast for energy.

Ingredients

- 1/2 cup rolled oats
- 1 cup almond milk (or your choice of milk)
- 1/2 cup mixed berries (strawberries, blueberries, raspberries)
- 2 tablespoons sliced almonds

- 1 tablespoon honey or maple syrup (optional, for sweetness)
- A pinch of cinnamon (optional, for flavor)

Instructions

- In a saucepan, combine the rolled oats and almond milk.

- Bring the mixture to a simmer over medium heat, stirring constantly.

- Cook until the oats are mushy and the oatmeal reaches your chosen consistency. This generally takes roughly 5-7 minutes.

- If you want sweetness, stir in honey or maple syrup and add a teaspoon of cinnamon for extra flavor.

- Pour the oatmeal into a bowl.

- Top with a large quantity of mixed berries and chopped almonds.

- Your oatmeal with berries and almonds is ready to treat you with a warm and nutritious breakfast.

Veggie and Cheese Breakfast Burrito

This scrumptious breakfast burrito is loaded with vegetables and cheese for a protein-packed and energetic start to your day.

Ingredients

- 1 whole wheat tortilla
- 2 large eggs
- 1/4 cup diced bell peppers
- 1/4 cup diced tomatoes
- 1/4 cup diced onions
- 1/4 cup shredded low-fat cheese
- Salt and pepper to taste
- Salsa or hot sauce (optional, for a kick)

Instructions

- In a bowl, beat the eggs and season with salt and pepper.

- Heat a non-stick skillet over medium heat and add a dash of oil.

- Add the diced bell peppers, tomatoes, and onions to the pan and sauté until they're soft.

- Pour the beaten eggs over the sautéed veggies and heat, turning regularly, until the eggs are cooked to your taste.

- Warm the whole wheat tortilla in a dry pan or microwave for a few seconds.

- Place the scrambled eggs and veggie mixture onto the tortilla.

- Sprinkle shredded low-fat cheese on top.

- If preferred, add a dash of salsa or spicy sauce for more flavor and spice.

- Fold the edges of the tortilla over the filling and wrap it up to form your breakfast burrito.

- Your vegetable and cheese breakfast burrito is ready for a tasty and pleasant morning meal.

Banana and Peanut Butter Breakfast Toast

This traditional combo of banana and peanut butter on whole-grain bread is easy, fast, and filled with energy. It's a wonderful option for hectic mornings.

Ingredients

- 1 slice of whole grain bread (or your choice of bread)
- 1 ripe banana, sliced

- 2 tablespoons natural peanut butter
- Honey or maple syrup (optional, for sweetness)
- A sprinkle of cinnamon (optional, for flavor)

Instructions

- Toast a piece of whole-grain bread to your chosen degree of crispiness.

- While the bread is toasting, slice the ripe banana.

- Once the bread is toasted, put the natural peanut butter on it.

- Arrange the banana slices on top of the peanut butter.

- If you like sweetness, sprinkle honey or maple syrup over the bananas. You may also add a sprinkling of cinnamon for added taste.

- Your banana and peanut butter breakfast toast is ready to present you with a delightful and energy-boosting morning.

Quinoa and Fruit Breakfast Bowl

Quinoa is a protein-rich grain that provides a terrific basis for a breakfast bowl. Top it with fresh fruit and a drizzle of honey for a wonderful and invigorating morning meal.

Ingredients

- 1/2 cup cooked quinoa
- 1/2 cup sliced fresh fruit (e.g., mango, kiwi, and pineapple)
- 1 tablespoon sliced almonds
- 1 tablespoon honey or maple syrup (optional, for sweetness)
- A pinch of cinnamon (optional, for flavor)

Instructions

- In a bowl, mix the cooked quinoa and cut fresh fruit.

- Top with sliced almonds.

- If you like sweetness, sprinkle honey or maple syrup over the quinoa and berries. You may also add a pinch of cinnamon for added taste.

- Your quinoa and fruit breakfast bowl is ready to offer you a protein-packed and refreshing start to your day.

Yogurt and Berry Parfait

This yogurt parfait is a simple and nutritious way to start your morning with a blast of flavors. The combination of yogurt, fresh berries, and granola gives a mix of protein, vitamins, and fiber.

Ingredients

- 1 cup low-fat Greek yogurt (or your choice of yogurt)
- 1/2 cup mixed berries (strawberries, blueberries, raspberries)
- 1/4 cup granola
- 1 tablespoon honey or maple syrup (optional, for sweetness)
- A sprinkle of cinnamon (optional, for flavor)

Instructions
- In a glass or dish, layer half of the low-fat Greek yogurt.

- Add a layer of mixed berries on top of the yogurt.

- Sprinkle granola over the berries.

- Drizzle honey or maple syrup over the granola for more sweetness, if preferred. You may also add a pinch of cinnamon for added taste.

- Layer the remaining low-fat Greek yogurt on top of the granola.

- Your yogurt and berry parfait are ready to offer you a protein-rich and enjoyable morning meal.

Veggie Breakfast Burrito Bowl

This breakfast burrito bowl is a pleasant and flavorful way to start your day with a selection of veggies, eggs, and the taste of your choice of salsa or spicy sauce.

Ingredients

- 2 large eggs

- 1/2 cup diced bell peppers (assorted colors)
- 1/4 cup diced tomatoes
- 1/4 cup diced onions
- 1/4 cup chopped spinach
- 1/4 cup black beans (canned or cooked)
- 1/4 cup shredded low-fat cheese
- Salt and pepper to taste
- Salsa or hot sauce (optional, for extra flavor)

Instructions

- In a bowl, beat the eggs and season with salt and pepper.

- In a pan over medium heat, sauté the chopped bell peppers, tomatoes, and onions until they're soft.

- Add the chopped spinach and simmer until it's wilted.

- Pour the beaten eggs into the skillet, and stir periodically while they cook.

- Once the eggs are nearly set, add the black beans and continue to cook, stirring, until the eggs are entirely cooked.

- Sprinkle shredded low-fat cheese on top and let it melt.

- Serve the vegetable breakfast burrito bowl in a bowl or dish.

- If preferred, add salsa or spicy sauce for more flavor and a kick.

- Your vegetable breakfast burrito bowl is ready for a full and invigorating morning.

Savory Breakfast Quinoa Bowl

This savory quinoa dish mixes the protein of quinoa with sautéed veggies and a poached egg for a delightful and full breakfast.

Ingredients

- 1/2 cup cooked quinoa
- 1/4 cup diced bell peppers (assorted colors)
- 1/4 cup diced zucchini
- 1/4 cup diced red onion
- 1/4 cup diced tomatoes
- 1 poached egg
- Salt and pepper to taste
- Fresh herbs (such as parsley or chives) for garnish

Instructions

- In a pan, sauté the chopped bell peppers, zucchini, red onion, and tomatoes until they're soft.

- In a bowl, mix the cooked quinoa with the sautéed veggies and season with salt and pepper.

- Poach one egg to your preference, keeping the yolk somewhat runny.

- Place the poached egg on top of the quinoa and veggie combination.

- Garnish with fresh herbs, such as parsley or chives.

- Your delicious breakfast quinoa dish is ready to serve you with a protein-packed and fulfilling morning.

Cottage Cheese and Fruit Bowl

This cottage cheese and fruit dish is a simple, protein-rich breakfast alternative with the sweetness of fresh fruit. It's a fast and refreshing option for your morning.

Ingredients

- 1 cup low-fat cottage cheese
- 1/2 cup sliced fresh fruit (e.g., pineapple, melon, or grapes)
- 1 tablespoon honey or maple syrup (optional, for sweetness)
- A sprinkle of cinnamon (optional, for flavor)

Instructions

- In a bowl, spoon out the low-fat cottage cheese.

- Top with sliced fresh fruit.

- If you like sweetness, sprinkle honey or maple syrup over the fruit. You may also add a pinch of cinnamon for added taste.

- Your cottage cheese and fruit dish is ready to offer you with a protein-rich and refreshing start to your day.

Blueberry and Almond Butter Oatmeal

Oatmeal is a popular breakfast choice, and this variant with blueberries and almond butter adds a wonderful touch. It's a healthful, energy-boosting way to start your day.

Ingredients

- 1/2 cup rolled oats
- 1 cup almond milk (or your choice of milk)
- 1/2 cup fresh or frozen blueberries
- 2 tablespoons almond butter
- Honey or maple syrup (optional, for sweetness)
- A sprinkle of sliced almonds (optional, for crunch)

Instructions

- In a saucepan, mix the rolled oats and almond milk.

- Bring the mixture to a simmer over medium heat, stirring regularly.

- Add the blueberries to the oats and continue to cook until the berries are mushy and the porridge reaches your preferred consistency. This normally takes approximately 5-7 minutes.

- Stir in almond butter for extra richness and taste.

- If you like sweetness, sprinkle honey or maple syrup over the oats.

- If you prefer a little crunch, put sliced almonds on top.

- Your blueberry and almond butter oatmeal is ready to serve you with a wholesome and comfortable morning.

Green Power Smoothie

This green power smoothie is rich with nutrients and gives a rush of energy to launch your day. It's a terrific method to sneak in more greens and superfoods into your diet.

Ingredients

- 1 cup fresh spinach
- 1/2 cup kale leaves (stems removed)
- 1/2 banana
- 1/2 cup pineapple chunks
- 1 tablespoon chia seeds
- 1 cup almond milk (or your choice of milk)
- 1 tablespoon honey or maple syrup (optional, for sweetness)

- A few ice cubes

Instructions

- Place the fresh spinach, kale, banana, pineapple pieces, chia seeds, almond milk, and ice cubes in a blender.

- Blend until you obtain a smooth and creamy consistency. If you like sweetness, you may add honey or maple syrup at this point.

- Pour the green power smoothie into a glass.

- Enjoy this nutrient-rich and invigorating smoothie to set your day off to a vivid start.

Berry and Quinoa Breakfast Bowl

This berry and quinoa breakfast dish is a delightful combination of nutritious grains and antioxidant-rich fruit. It's a fantastic option for individuals who want a hearty start to their day.

Ingredients

- 1/2 cup cooked quinoa
- 1/2 cup mixed berries (strawberries, blueberries, raspberries)
- 1 tablespoon sliced almonds
- 1 tablespoon honey or maple syrup (optional, for sweetness)
- A sprinkle of cinnamon (optional, for flavor)

Instructions

- In a bowl, combine the cooked quinoa and mixed berries.

- Top with sliced almonds.

- If you like sweetness, sprinkle honey or maple syrup over the quinoa and berries.

You may also add a pinch of cinnamon for added taste.

- Your berry and quinoa breakfast bowl is ready to serve you a healthy and energy-boosting morning.

Chapter 5

Lunches to Fuel Your Day

Balanced and Delicious Lunch Ideas
Lunch is a chance to recharge your body, continue supporting your prostate health, and have a tasty and balanced meal. In this part, we'll examine several lunch choices that are not only tasty but also intended to give you the required nutrients to keep your energy levels high and your prostate in excellent condition.

Grilled Chicken Salad

Grilled chicken salad is a popular lunch choice that mixes healthy protein with a variety of veggies and a tasty dressing. It's a meal that finds a wonderful balance between flavor and nutrition.

Ingredients

- 4 oz grilled chicken breast, sliced
- Mixed salad greens (e.g., spinach, arugula, and romaine)
- Cherry tomatoes, halved
- Cucumber slices
- Red onion slices
- A sprinkle of feta cheese (optional)
- Balsamic vinaigrette dressing

Instructions

- Arrange the mixed salad greens on a platter or in a dish.

- Add the grilled chicken breast pieces on top of the greens.

- Scatter cherry tomatoes, cucumber slices, and red onion slices over the salad.

- If preferred, put a piece of feta cheese on top for more flavor.

- Drizzle the balsamic vinaigrette dressing over the salad shortly before serving.

- Your grilled chicken salad is ready to offer you with a well-balanced and tasty meal.

Quinoa and Vegetable Bowl

A quinoa and vegetable bowl is a healthy, plant-based lunch choice that blends healthful grains with a vibrant variety of veggies. It's an excellent alternative for individuals who prefer vegetarian meals.

Ingredients

- 1/2 cup cooked quinoa

- Mixed vegetables (e.g., bell peppers, zucchini, carrots, and broccoli), diced and roasted
- Chickpeas, rinsed and drained
- Feta cheese or crumbled goat cheese (optional)
- Hummus or tahini dressing

Instructions

- In a bowl, combine the cooked quinoa and the roasted mixed veggies.

- Add chickpeas to the dish for extra protein.

- If preferred, put feta cheese or crumbled goat cheese over top for more taste.

- Drizzle hummus or tahini dressing over the dish shortly before serving.

- Your quinoa and veggie bowl is ready to offer you a well-balanced and pleasant meal.

Salmon and Quinoa Salad

This salmon and quinoa salad is not only tasty but also full of omega-3 fatty acids and protein, making it a perfect option for a prostate-healthy lunch.

Ingredients

- 4 oz grilled or baked salmon
- 1/2 cup cooked quinoa
- Mixed salad greens (e.g., spinach, arugula, and romaine)
- Sliced red bell pepper
- Sliced cucumber
- Lemon vinaigrette dressing

Instructions

- Place the mixed salad greens on a platter or in a dish.

- Add the cooked quinoa on top of the greens.

- Place the grilled or baked fish atop the quinoa.

- Scatter sliced red bell pepper and cucumber over the salad.

- Drizzle lemon vinaigrette dressing over the salad shortly before serving.

- Your salmon and quinoa salad is ready to serve you with a well-balanced and tasty meal.

Mediterranean Chickpea Wrap

This Mediterranean chickpea wrap is a tasty and plant-based lunch choice loaded with the richness of chickpeas, veggies, and a zesty tahini sauce.

Ingredients

- 1 whole wheat or spinach wrap
- 1 cup canned chickpeas, rinsed and drained
- Diced cucumber
- Sliced cherry tomatoes
- Chopped red onion
- Fresh parsley leaves
- Tahini sauce (tahini, lemon juice, and garlic)

Instructions

- Warm the whole wheat or spinach wrap, if preferred.

- In a dish, combine the canned chickpeas with diced cucumber, sliced cherry tomatoes, chopped red onion, and fresh parsley leaves.

- Drizzle the tahini sauce over the chickpea mixture and toss to coat.

- Spoon the chickpea mixture onto the wrap.

- Fold the edges of the wrap over the contents and roll it up to form your Mediterranean chickpea wrap.

- Your wrap is ready to offer you a wonderful and balanced meal.

Turkey and Avocado Sandwich

A turkey and avocado sandwich is a traditional option for a filling and protein-rich lunch that's simple to make and filled with flavor.

Ingredients

- Whole grain bread or a whole wheat wrap
- Sliced turkey breast
- Sliced avocado
- Lettuce leaves

- Sliced tomato
- Dijon mustard or low-fat mayo (optional)
- A sprinkle of black pepper

Instructions

- If using bread, toast it to your satisfaction.

- Layer sliced turkey breast on the bread or wrap.

- Add slices of ripe avocado, lettuce leaves, and sliced tomato.

- If preferred, add Dijon mustard or low-fat mayo for extra taste.

- Sprinkle a dab of black pepper for a last touch.

- Your turkey and avocado sandwich is ready to offer you with a healthy and tasty meal.

Veggie and Brown Rice Stir-Fry

A veggie and brown rice stir-fry is a healthful and adaptable lunch choice that enables you to mix a range of veggies and lean protein options.

Ingredients

- Cooked brown rice
- Mixed vegetables (e.g., broccoli, bell peppers, snap peas, and carrots), chopped
- Tofu, tempeh, or skinless chicken breast, diced
- Low-sodium soy sauce or teriyaki sauce
- Sliced green onions
- Sesame seeds (optional)

Instructions

- In a large skillet or wok, heat a tiny quantity of oil over medium-high heat.

- Add the chopped tofu, tempeh, or skinless chicken breast and heat until it's nearly done.

- Add the chopped mixed veggies and continue to stir-fry until they're tender-crisp.

- Mix in cooked brown rice.

- Drizzle low-sodium soy sauce or teriyaki sauce over the stir-fry and toss to coat.

- Serve the stir-fry in a dish, topped with sliced green onions and sesame seeds, if preferred.

- Your vegetable and brown rice stir-fry is ready to serve you with a healthy and delectable meal.

Spinach and Feta Stuffed Chicken Breast

This spinach and feta-filled chicken breast is a tasty and protein-packed lunch choice that's both impressive and quick to cook.

Ingredients

- 1 boneless, skinless chicken breast
- 1 cup fresh spinach leaves
- 2 tablespoons crumbled feta cheese
- Salt and pepper to taste
- Olive oil for cooking

Instructions

- Preheat your oven to 375°F (190°C).

- Butterfly the chicken breast by cutting it in half horizontally, leaving one edge uncut. Open the chicken breast like a book.

- Lay the chicken breast flat and lay the fresh spinach leaves and crumbled feta cheese on one side of the chicken.

- Fold the opposite side of the chicken breast over the filling to make a filled chicken breast.

- Season both sides of the chicken with salt and pepper.

- Heat a small quantity of olive oil in an oven-safe skillet over medium-high heat.

- Place the filled chicken breast in the pan and cook for 2-3 minutes on each side until it's well browned.

- Transfer the pan to the preheated oven and bake for approximately 15-20 minutes, or until the chicken is cooked through and no longer pink in the middle.

- Let it rest for a few minutes before slicing and serving.

- Your spinach and feta-filled chicken breast is ready to offer you a tasty and protein-rich meal.

Greek Salad with Grilled Shrimp

This Greek salad with grilled shrimp is a light and refreshing lunch choice that mixes the tastes of the Mediterranean with a dose of nutritious protein.

Ingredients

- Grilled shrimp (4-6 shrimp per serving)
- Mixed salad greens (e.g., romaine, red leaf, and green leaf)
- Cucumber slices
- Cherry tomatoes, halved
- Kalamata olives
- Crumbled feta cheese

- Greek salad dressing

Instructions

- Prepare the grilled shrimp by marinating them in your choice of seasonings and grilling until they're done.

- Arrange mixed salad greens on a dish or in a bowl.

- Add grilled shrimp, cucumber slices, cherry tomatoes, Kalamata olives, and crumbled feta cheese.

- Drizzle Greek salad dressing over the salad shortly before serving.

- Your Greek salad with grilled shrimp is ready to give you a pleasant and balanced meal.

Tuna and White Bean Salad

Tuna and white bean salad is a protein-rich and substantial lunch choice that's quick to make and loaded with tastes and textures.

Ingredients

- Canned tuna in water, drained
- Canned white beans, rinsed and drained
- Red onion, finely chopped
- Fresh parsley leaves, chopped
- Lemon juice
- Olive oil
- Salt and pepper to taste

Instructions

- In a dish, mix the canned tuna, canned white beans, chopped red onion, and chopped fresh parsley leaves.

- Drizzle lemon juice and olive oil over the mixture.

- Season with salt and pepper, and toss to mix.

- Your tuna and white bean salad is ready to offer you a tasty and protein-packed lunch.

Mango and Black Bean Quinoa Salad

This mango and black bean quinoa salad is a colorful and nutrient-rich lunch choice that mixes the sweetness of mango with the protein of black beans and quinoa.

Ingredients

- Cooked quinoa
- Canned black beans, rinsed and drained
- Diced ripe mango
- Diced red bell pepper
- Red onion, finely chopped
- Fresh cilantro leaves, chopped
- Lime juice

- Olive oil
- Salt and pepper to taste

Instructions

- In a bowl, add cooked quinoa, canned black beans, diced ripe mango, diced red bell pepper, and finely sliced red onion.

- Drizzle lime juice and olive oil over the mixture.

- Season with salt and pepper, and toss to mix.

- Garnish with chopped fresh cilantro leaves.

- Your mango and black bean quinoa salad is ready to offer you a healthy and delightful meal.

Mushroom and Spinach Stuffed Pita

This mushroom and spinach-filled pita is a wonderful vegetarian lunch alternative that's packed with earthy flavors and lush greens.

Ingredients

- Whole wheat pita bread
- Sliced mushrooms
- Fresh spinach leaves
- Red onion, finely chopped
- Crumbled goat cheese or feta cheese (optional)
- Olive oil for cooking
- Balsamic vinaigrette dressing

Instructions

- Heat a small quantity of olive oil in a pan over medium-high heat.

- Add the sliced mushrooms and sauté until they're soft.

- Add fresh spinach leaves and diced red onion to the pan and heat until the spinach wilts.

- If preferred, add crumbled goat cheese or feta cheese over the mixture for more taste.

- Warm the whole wheat pita bread, if preferred.

- Spoon the mushroom and spinach mixture into the pita.

- Drizzle balsamic vinaigrette dressing shortly before serving.

- Your mushroom and spinach-loaded pita is ready to give you a wonderful and balanced meal.

Veggie and Quinoa Wrap

A veggie and quinoa wrap is a healthful and plant-based lunch choice loaded with colorful veggies and protein-packed quinoa.

Ingredients

- Whole wheat or spinach wrap
- Cooked quinoa
- Sliced bell peppers (assorted colors)
- Sliced cucumber
- Sliced tomatoes
- Sliced red onion
- Fresh basil leaves
- Hummus or tahini dressing

Instructions

- Warm the whole wheat or spinach wrap, if preferred.

- Spread a thick amount of cooked quinoa over the wrap.

- Arrange sliced bell peppers, cucumber, tomatoes, and red onion on top of the quinoa.

- Add fresh basil leaves for a punch of flavor.

- Drizzle hummus or tahini dressing over the wrap shortly before serving.

- Your vegetable and quinoa wrap is ready to give you a nutritious and tasty meal.

Egg Salad Lettuce Wraps

Egg salad lettuce wraps give a light and protein-rich lunch alternative. They're a low-carb alternative to classic sandwiches, enabling you to experience the creamy richness of egg salad with a healthy twist.

Ingredients

- Hard-boiled eggs, chopped
- Greek yogurt or low-fat mayonnaise
- Dijon mustard
- Chopped celery
- Chopped green onions
- Salt and pepper to taste
- Large lettuce leaves (e.g., iceberg or butter lettuce)

Instructions

- In a bowl, combine the chopped hard-boiled eggs, Greek yogurt or low-fat mayonnaise, and Dijon mustard. Adjust the amount to reach your desired creaminess.

- Add chopped celery and green onions to the mixture.

- Season with salt and pepper, and mix well.

- Spoon the egg salad onto large lettuce leaves.

- Roll the lettuce leaves to create egg salad lettuce wraps.

- Your egg salad lettuce wraps are ready to provide you with a light and protein-packed lunch.

Caprese Salad with Grilled Chicken

A Caprese salad with grilled chicken is a classic lunch option that combines the freshness of tomatoes and basil with the protein of grilled chicken.

Ingredients

- Grilled chicken breast, sliced
- Sliced tomatoes
- Fresh basil leaves
- Fresh mozzarella cheese, sliced

- Balsamic glaze
- Olive oil
- Salt and pepper to taste

Instructions

- Arrange the grilled chicken breast pieces, sliced tomatoes, fresh basil leaves, and sliced fresh mozzarella cheese on a platter.

- Drizzle balsamic glaze and olive oil over the salad.

- Season with salt and pepper.

- Your Caprese salad with grilled chicken is ready to offer you a fresh and protein-rich meal.

Chicken Caesar Salad

The traditional Chicken Caesar salad is a filling and delicious lunch choice that blends grilled chicken with crisp romaine lettuce, croutons, and a creamy Caesar dressing.

Ingredients

- Grilled chicken breast, sliced
- Romaine lettuce leaves
- Croutons
- Shredded Parmesan cheese
- Caesar dressing

Instructions

- Arrange the grilled chicken breast pieces, romaine lettuce leaves, croutons, and grated Parmesan cheese on a dish.

- Drizzle Caesar dressing over the salad.

- Toss the salad to coat the ingredients equally.

- Your Chicken Caesar salad is ready to offer you a healthy and pleasant meal.

Turkey and Avocado Wrap

The turkey and avocado wrap is a filling and protein-rich lunch choice that mixes the lean protein of turkey with the smoothness of avocado.

Ingredients

- Whole wheat or spinach wrap
- Sliced turkey breast
- Sliced avocado
- Lettuce leaves
- Sliced tomato
- Dijon mustard or low-fat mayo (optional)
- A sprinkle of black pepper

Instructions

- Warm the whole wheat or spinach wrap, if preferred.

- Layer sliced turkey breast on the wrap.

- Add slices of ripe avocado, lettuce leaves, and sliced tomato.

- If preferred, add Dijon mustard or low-fat mayo for extra taste.

- Sprinkle a dab of black pepper for a last touch.

- Your turkey and avocado wrap is ready to serve you a full and fulfilling meal.

Chapter 6

Dinner Delights

Flavorful Dinners for Prostate Health
Dinner is a time to relax and eat a well-balanced meal that not only pleases your taste buds but also feeds your body, including your prostate health. In this part, we'll examine a range of supper dishes that are meant to be both savory and supportive of prostate health.

Grilled Salmon with Lemon and Dill

Grilled salmon with lemon and dill is a traditional supper choice that's not only tasty but also high in omega-3 fatty acids, which may enhance prostate health.

Ingredients

- Salmon fillet
- Lemon slices
- Fresh dill
- Olive oil
- Salt and pepper to taste

Instructions

- Preheat your grill to medium-high heat.

- Season the salmon fillet with olive oil, salt, and pepper.

- Place lemon slices and fresh dill on top of the salmon.

- Grill the salmon for approximately 4-5 minutes on each side, or until it flakes easily with a fork.

- Your grilled salmon with lemon and dill is ready to present you with a tasty and prostate-friendly supper.

Quinoa-stuffed bell Peppers

Quinoa-stuffed bell peppers are a colorful and healthy supper alternative that includes quinoa, lean protein, and a variety of veggies.

Ingredients

- Bell peppers (red, green, or yellow)
- Cooked quinoa
- Ground turkey or lean ground beef (or meat substitute)
- Diced tomatoes
- Chopped onions
- Garlic, minced
- Tomato sauce
- Italian seasoning
- Salt and pepper to taste

Instructions

- Preheat your oven to 350°F (175°C).

- Cut the tops off the bell peppers and remove the seeds and membranes.

- In a skillet, brown the ground turkey or lean ground beef. If you want a vegetarian version, sauté meat replacement as required.

- Add diced tomatoes, chopped onions, and minced garlic to the pan and heat until the veggies are soft.

- Mix in cooked quinoa, tomato sauce, Italian seasoning, salt, and pepper.

- Stuff the bell peppers with the quinoa and beef mixture.

- Place the filled bell peppers in a baking tray and cover with aluminum foil.

- Bake for approximately 25-30 minutes, or until the peppers are cooked.

- Your quinoa-stuffed bell peppers are ready to serve you with a colorful and prostate-friendly meal.

Baked Chicken with Roasted Vegetables

Baked chicken with roasted vegetables is a filling supper choice that mixes lean protein with a variety of colorful veggies, offering a range of critical elements.

Ingredients

- Boneless, skinless chicken breast or thigh
- Mixed vegetables (e.g., carrots, broccoli, bell peppers, and zucchini), chopped
- Olive oil

- Garlic powder
- Italian seasoning
- Salt and pepper to taste

Instructions

- Preheat your oven to 375°F (190°C).

- In a large bowl, combine the mixed veggies with olive oil, garlic powder, Italian seasoning, salt, and pepper.

- Place the chicken and seasoned veggies on a baking sheet.

- Bake for approximately 25-30 minutes, or until the chicken is cooked through and the veggies are soft.

- Your cooked chicken with roasted veggies is ready to serve you with a substantial and prostate-friendly supper.

Spaghetti Squash with Turkey Bolognese

Spaghetti squash with turkey Bolognese is a low-carb and tasty meal alternative that swaps regular pasta with roasted spaghetti squash.

Ingredients

- Spaghetti squash
- Ground turkey
- Diced tomatoes
- Tomato sauce
- Chopped onions
- Garlic, minced
- Italian seasoning
- Salt and pepper to taste
- Fresh basil leaves

Instructions

- Preheat your oven to 375°F (190°C).

- Cut the spaghetti squash in half lengthwise and remove the seeds.

- Place the squash halves, cut side down, on a baking sheet and roast for approximately 40 minutes, or until the flesh is soft.

- While the squash is roasting, brown the ground turkey in a pan.

- Add diced tomatoes, tomato sauce, chopped onions, minced garlic, Italian seasoning, salt, and pepper to the pan.

- Simmer the sauce for approximately 15-20 minutes, allowing the flavors to mingle.

- Use a fork to scrape the baked spaghetti squash flesh into "noodles."

- Serve the turkey Bolognese sauce over the spaghetti squash and decorate with fresh basil leaves.

- Your spaghetti squash with turkey Bolognese is ready to serve you with a tasty and prostate-friendly meal.

Vegetarian Chili

Vegetarian chili is a substantial and healthful meal choice that mixes a range of veggies and beans with fragrant spices.

Ingredients

- Canned kidney beans, drained and rinsed
- Canned black beans, drained and rinsed
- Canned chickpeas, drained and rinsed
- Diced tomatoes
- Chopped onions
- Bell peppers, diced
- Corn kernels
- Vegetable broth
- Chili powder, cumin, and paprika
- Salt and pepper to taste

Instructions

- In a large saucepan, sauté the chopped onions and diced bell peppers until they're soft.

- Add chopped tomatoes, kidney beans, black beans, chickpeas, and corn kernels to the saucepan.

- Stir in vegetable broth, chili powder, cumin, paprika, salt, and pepper.

- Simmer the chili for approximately 20-25 minutes to allow the flavors to combine and the veggies to soften.

- Your vegetarian chili is ready to serve you with a substantial and prostate-friendly meal.

Grilled Vegetable and Quinoa Bowl

A grilled vegetable and quinoa bowl is a tasty and plant-based supper option that's filled with nutrient-rich veggies and protein-packed quinoa.

Ingredients

- Cooked quinoa
- Mixed vegetables (e.g., zucchini, eggplant, bell peppers, and red onion), sliced
- Olive oil
- Balsamic vinegar
- Garlic, minced
- Fresh basil leaves
- Salt and pepper to taste

Instructions

- Preheat your grill to medium-high heat.

- Toss the sliced mixed veggies with olive oil, balsamic vinegar, minced garlic, salt, and pepper.

- Grill the veggies for approximately 3-4 minutes on each side, or until they're cooked and have grill marks.

- Serve the grilled veggies over a bed of cooked quinoa and decorate with fresh basil leaves.

- Your grilled veggie and quinoa dish is ready to offer you a tasty and prostate-friendly meal.

Lentil and Vegetable Stir-Fry

Lentil and vegetable stir-fry is a healthy and adaptable meal choice that enables you to mix protein-rich lentils with a range of colorful veggies.

Ingredients

- Cooked lentils
- Mixed vegetables (e.g., broccoli, bell peppers, snap peas, and carrots), chopped
- Low-sodium soy sauce or teriyaki sauce
- Sliced green onions
- Sesame seeds (optional)

Instructions

- In a large skillet or wok, heat a tiny quantity of oil over medium-high heat.

- Add the chopped mixed veggies and stir-fry until they're tender-crisp.

- Mix in cooked lentils.

- Drizzle low-sodium soy sauce or teriyaki sauce over the stir-fry and toss to coat.

- Serve the lentil and vegetable stir-fry in a dish, topped with sliced green onions and sesame seeds, if preferred.

- Your lentil and vegetable stir-fry is ready to give you a nutrient-rich and prostate-friendly meal.

Baked Sweet Potato with Chickpea Curry

Baked sweet potato with chickpea curry is a filling and nutrient-packed meal choice that mixes the sweetness of sweet potatoes with the richness of chickpea curry.

Ingredients

- Sweet potatoes
- Canned chickpeas, drained and rinsed
- Diced tomatoes
- Chopped onions
- Garlic, minced
- Curry powder and cumin

- Salt and pepper to taste
- Fresh cilantro leaves

Instructions

- Preheat your oven to 400°F (200°C).

- Pierce the sweet potatoes with a fork and lay them on a baking pan.

- Bake for approximately 45-50 minutes, or until the sweet potatoes are soft.

- While the sweet potatoes are roasting, sauté the chopped onions and minced garlic until they're soft.

- Add diced tomatoes, canned chickpeas, curry powder, cumin, salt, and pepper to the pan.

- Simmer the chickpea curry for around 15-20 minutes.

- Slice open the roasted sweet potatoes and fill them with the chickpea curry.

- Garnish with fresh cilantro leaves.

- Your roasted sweet potato with chickpea curry is ready to present you with a tasty and prostate-friendly meal.

Mushroom and Spinach Stuffed Chicken

Mushroom and spinach-filled chicken is a tasty and protein-rich meal choice that's both elegant and quick to cook.

Ingredients

- Boneless, skinless chicken breast
- Sliced mushrooms
- Fresh spinach leaves
- Red onion, finely chopped
- Crumbled goat cheese or feta cheese (optional)

- Olive oil for cooking
- Balsamic glaze

Instructions

- Preheat your oven to 375°F (190°C).

- Butterfly the chicken breast by cutting it in half horizontally, leaving one edge uncut. Open the chicken breast like a book.

- Lay the chicken breast flat and arrange the sliced mushrooms, fresh spinach leaves, and chopped red onion on one side of the chicken.

- If preferred, add crumbled goat cheese or feta cheese over the mixture for more taste.

- Fold the opposite side of the chicken breast over the filling to make a filled chicken breast.

- Season with salt and pepper.

- Heat a small quantity of olive oil in an oven-safe skillet over medium-high heat.

- Place the filled chicken breast in the pan and cook for 2-3 minutes on each side until it's well browned.

- Transfer the pan to the preheated oven and bake for approximately 15-20 minutes, or until the chicken is cooked through and no longer pink in the middle.

- Drizzle balsamic glaze over the chicken right before serving.

- Your mushroom and spinach-filled chicken is ready to serve you with a delectable and prostate-friendly meal.

Grilled Vegetable and Quinoa Bowl

A grilled vegetable and quinoa bowl is a tasty and plant-based supper option that's filled with nutrient-rich veggies and protein-packed quinoa.

Ingredients

- Cooked quinoa
- Mixed vegetables (e.g., zucchini, eggplant, bell peppers, and red onion), sliced
- Olive oil
- Balsamic vinegar
- Garlic, minced
- Fresh basil leaves
- Salt and pepper to taste

Instructions

- Preheat your grill to medium-high heat.

- Toss the sliced mixed veggies with olive oil, balsamic vinegar, minced garlic, salt, and pepper.

- Grill the veggies for approximately 3-4 minutes on each side, or until they're cooked and have grill marks.

- Serve the grilled veggies over a bed of cooked quinoa and decorate with fresh basil leaves.

- Your grilled veggie and quinoa dish is ready to offer you with a tasty and prostate-friendly meal.

Eggplant Parmesan

Eggplant Parmesan is a filling and delicious supper choice that mixes soft eggplant slices with rich tomato sauce and melting cheese.

Ingredients

- Eggplant, thinly sliced
- Bread crumbs (you can use whole wheat or gluten-free for a healthier option)
- Egg whites (for breading)
- Tomato sauce (low-sodium or homemade)
- Mozzarella cheese, shredded
- Parmesan cheese, grated
- Fresh basil leaves
- Olive oil
- Salt and pepper to taste

Instructions

- Preheat your oven to 375°F (190°C).

- Dip each eggplant slice in egg whites, then cover with bread crumbs.

- Heat a tiny quantity of olive oil in a pan over medium-high heat.

- Sauté the breaded eggplant slices until they're golden brown.

- In a baking dish, stack the sautéed eggplant pieces, tomato sauce, mozzarella cheese, Parmesan cheese, and fresh basil leaves.

- Repeat the stacking until you've used all the ingredients.

- Bake for approximately 20-25 minutes, or until the cheese is melted and bubbling.

- Your eggplant Parmesan is ready to serve you with a delicious and prostate-friendly meal.

Sesame-Ginger Tofu Stir-Fry

Sesame-ginger tofu stir-fry is a plant-based supper alternative that's overflowing with flavors and filled with protein from tofu.

Ingredients

- Extra-firm tofu, cubed
- Mixed vegetables (e.g., broccoli, bell peppers, snap peas, and carrots), chopped
- Low-sodium soy sauce
- Sesame oil
- Fresh ginger, minced
- Garlic, minced
- Sesame seeds
- Green onions, sliced
- Brown rice or quinoa (for serving)

Instructions

- In a large skillet or wok, heat a tiny quantity of oil over medium-high heat.

- Add the cubed tofu and stir-fry until it's lightly browned on both sides.

- Remove the tofu from the skillet.

- In the same pan, add a touch more oil if required and sauté the chopped mixed veggies, fresh ginger, and minced garlic until they're tender-crisp.

- Add the cooked tofu back to the skillet.

- Drizzle low-sodium soy sauce and sesame oil over the stir-fry and toss to coat.

- Serve the sesame-ginger tofu stir-fry over brown rice or quinoa, topped with sesame seeds and sliced green onions.

- Your sesame-ginger tofu stir-fry is ready to give you a tasty and prostate-friendly meal.

Salmon and Asparagus Foil Pack

Salmon and asparagus foil packets are a simple and tasty meal alternative that keeps the flavors sealed in and reduces cleaning.

Ingredients

- Salmon fillet
- Asparagus spears
- Lemon slices
- Fresh dill
- Olive oil
- Salt and pepper to taste

Instructions

- Preheat your oven to 375°F (190°C).

- Place a piece of aluminum foil on a baking pan.

- Lay the salmon fillet on the foil.

- Arrange asparagus spears, lemon slices, and fresh dill around the fish.

- Drizzle olive oil over the salmon and asparagus, and season with salt and pepper.

- Fold the foil to make a package, sealing the edges securely.

- Bake for approximately 15-20 minutes, or until the salmon flakes easily with a fork.

- Your salmon and asparagus foil pack is ready to serve you with an easy and prostate-friendly supper.

Chickpea and Vegetable Curry

Chickpea and vegetable curry is a tasty and plant-based supper option that mixes chickpeas with a variety of vegetables in a creamy and fragrant sauce.

Ingredients

- Cooked chickpeas
- Mixed vegetables (e.g., bell peppers, cauliflower, carrots, and peas)
- Chopped onions

- Garlic, minced
- Curry powder, cumin, and coriander
- Coconut milk
- Salt and pepper to taste
- Fresh cilantro leaves

Instructions

- In a large saucepan, sauté the chopped onions and minced garlic until they're soft.

- Add mixed veggies and stir-fry until they're slightly softened.

- Mix in cooked chickpeas, curry powder, cumin, coriander, salt, and pepper.

- Pour in coconut milk and boil for around 10-15 minutes, allowing the flavors to mingle.

- Serve the chickpea and vegetable stew over rice, quinoa, or whole wheat couscous, topped with fresh cilantro leaves.

- Your chickpea and vegetable curry is ready to offer you a tasty and prostate-friendly meal.

Quinoa and Black Bean Skillet

The quinoa and black bean skillet is a one-pot miracle that's both easy and filled with nutrition.

Ingredients

- Cooked quinoa
- Black beans, drained and rinsed
- Diced tomatoes
- Chopped onions
- Garlic, minced
- Chili powder, cumin, and paprika
- Fresh cilantro leaves
- Salt and pepper to taste

Instructions

- In a large pan, sauté the chopped onions and minced garlic until they're soft.

- Add chopped tomatoes, black beans, cooked quinoa, chili powder, cumin, paprika, salt, and pepper.

- Simmer for around 10-15 minutes, allowing the flavors to mingle.

- Garnish with fresh cilantro leaves.

- Your quinoa and black bean skillet is ready to give you a simple and prostate-friendly meal.

Grilled Portobello Mushrooms

Grilled Portobello mushrooms are a simple and delectable supper choice that's both adaptable and delicious.

Ingredients

- Portobello mushrooms
- Balsamic vinegar
- Olive oil
- Fresh rosemary and thyme leaves
- Salt and pepper to taste

Instructions

- Preheat your grill to medium-high heat.

- In a dish, combine balsamic vinegar, olive oil, fresh rosemary, thyme, salt, and pepper.

- Brush the Portobello mushrooms with the mixture.

- Grill the mushrooms for approximately 4-5 minutes on each side, or until they're soft.

- Your grilled Portobello mushrooms are ready to serve you with an easy and prostate-friendly meal.

Chapter 7

Snacks and Sides

Prostate-Friendly Snack Ideas
Snacking may be a vital part of your daily eating routine, and it's a chance to make prostate-friendly choices that are both tasty and enjoyable. In this part, we'll examine several snack choices meant to promote your prostate health.

1. Mixed Nuts

Nuts are a terrific snack choice that contains healthy fats and plant-based protein. They are also high in antioxidants, which are helpful for prostate health. A handful of mixed nuts like almonds, walnuts, and pistachios helps keep your energy up and your prostate in excellent health.

2. Greek Yogurt with Berries

Greek yogurt is packed with protein, and when mixed with antioxidant-rich berries like blueberries or strawberries, it creates a delectable and prostate-friendly snack. The combination of protein and antioxidants enhances general well-being, including prostate health.

3. Carrot and Hummus

Carrots are a wonderful source of vitamins and minerals, while hummus delivers plant-based protein. Together, they make for a filling snack that's high in fiber and minerals. Carrot and hummus sticks are not only tasty but also fantastic for your prostate.

4. Edamame

Edamame, young soybeans, is a nutrient-dense snack filled with plant-based protein and fiber. They also include substances like isoflavones, which are connected with prostate health. Steamed edamame with a sprinkling of sea salt makes for a delightful and healthful snack.

5. Celery with Almond Butter

Celery sticks coupled with almond butter offer a balanced and crispy snack. Almond butter delivers healthful fats and protein, while celery is a hydrating and low-calorie plant. This combo is not only pleasant but also helpful for your prostate health.

6. Chia Pudding

Chia pudding is a diverse and healthful snack that's easy to make. Chia seeds are abundant in fiber, omega-3 fatty acids, and plant-based protein. You may prepare a chia pudding by combining chia seeds with your choice of milk (e.g., almond, soy, or coconut) and sweetening it with a touch of honey or maple syrup. Let it rest in the refrigerator to thicken, then top it with fresh fruits or nuts for added taste and prostate health benefits.

7. Sliced Avocado with Whole Grain Crackers

Avocado is a source of healthful monounsaturated fats, and it mixes nicely with whole-grain crackers. This combination is not only tasty but also contains healthy fats and fiber, which are beneficial for your prostate.

8. Berries with Dark Chocolate

Berries like blueberries and strawberries are filled with antioxidants that may boost prostate health. Dark chocolate with a high cocoa content also includes antioxidants. Pairing a tiny portion of dark chocolate with a bowl of fresh fruit produces a pleasant and prostate-friendly snack.

9. Cottage Cheese with Pineapple

Cottage cheese is a protein-rich snack that mixes wonderfully with the sweet and acidic taste of pineapple. It's a balanced and nutrient-dense alternative that may assist your prostate health while gratifying your taste senses.

10. Sliced Cucumber with Tzatziki

Cucumber slices coupled with tzatziki, a yogurt-based dip, make for a pleasant and hydrated snack. Cucumbers are low in calories and rich in water content, while tzatziki delivers protein and probiotics that may be excellent for your digestive system and general health.

11. Quinoa Salad

Quinoa salad is a flexible and pleasant snack that can be made in advance and consumed throughout the day. You may prepare a prostate-friendly quinoa salad by mixing cooked quinoa with chopped vegetables, herbs, and a mild vinaigrette. It's a nutrient-dense food that contains fiber, plant-based protein, and vitamins.

12. Sliced Apple with Almond Butter

Apples are a significant source of fiber and antioxidants. When you slice an apple and couple it with almond butter, you get a combination of natural sweetness and healthy fats. This food is not only tasty but also helpful for prostate health.

13. Whole Grain Popcorn

Whole grain popcorn is a fiber-rich and low-calorie snack that may be a delightful option when you need something crunchy. Opt for air-popped popcorn or mildly seasoned types to keep it prostate-friendly.

14. Green Smoothie

A green smoothie is a healthful snack that may be filled with vegetables and fruits. You may combine items like spinach, kale, banana, and almond milk to produce a delicious and vitamin-packed drink. The antioxidants from greens and fruits might help your prostate health.

15. Walnut and Date Energy Balls

Homemade walnut and date energy balls are a quick and energy-boosting snack. Walnuts are rich in healthful fats and protein, while dates give natural sweetness. Simply combine these ingredients and mold them into little energy balls for a fast and prostate-friendly snack.

16. Sliced Bell Peppers with Guacamole

Bell peppers, particularly the colorful ones, are rich in antioxidants and vitamin C. Sliced bell peppers coupled with guacamole, created from mashed avocado, give a crisp and creamy mix that's both tasty and supportive of your prostate health.

17. Hard-Boiled Eggs

Hard-boiled eggs are a protein-packed snack that's simple to prepare in advance and have on hand. They are a fantastic source of protein, vitamins, and minerals, making them a diverse and prostate-friendly alternative.

18. Cottage Cheese with Sliced Tomatoes

Cottage cheese is a protein-rich alternative that works beautifully with sliced tomatoes. Tomatoes include lycopene, an antioxidant related to prostate health. This snack is not only delightful but also helpful for your well-being.

These snack options provide a range of alternatives to keep you full between meals while supporting your prostate health. Whether you like the simplicity of whole grain popcorn, the nutrient-packed green smoothie, or the handmade walnut and date energy balls, each snack is meant to be both handy and helpful for your general well-being.

Nutrient-Packed Side Dishes

In addition to prostate-friendly snacks, integrating nutrient-packed side dishes into your meals will further increase your general health and well-being. Here are some tasty and healthful side dish ideas:

1. Steamed Broccoli with Garlic and Lemon

Steamed broccoli is a healthful side dish, and when you add a bit of garlic and a splash of lemon, it becomes even more delectable. Broccoli is rich in antioxidants and fiber, making it a fantastic option for your prostate health.

2. Quinoa and Vegetable Stir-Fry

Quinoa is a protein-rich grain that goes nicely with a range of bright veggies. A quinoa and veggie stir-fry is a nutrient-packed side meal that's not only tasty but also supportive of your general well-being.

3. Mixed Berry Salad

A mixed berry salad mixes diverse berries such as blueberries, strawberries, and raspberries. Berries are packed with antioxidants and vitamins, making this side dish a delightful and healthy complement to your meals.

4. Cauliflower Mash

Cauliflower mash is a nutritious alternative to regular mashed potatoes. Cauliflower is a cruciferous vegetable that's renowned for its potential advantages for prostate health. Mashed cauliflower is a creamy and pleasant side dish that's lower in carbohydrates and calories.

5. Spinach and Strawberry Salad

Spinach and strawberry salad is a lovely blend of lush greens and sweet strawberries. Spinach is a source of vitamins and minerals, while strawberries are rich in antioxidants. A little vinaigrette may make this side dish even more enticing.

6. Roasted Brussels Sprouts

Roasted Brussels sprouts are a tasty side dish that's strong in fiber and minerals. The roasting procedure brings out their inherent sweetness and makes them a terrific complement to your meals.

7. Brown Rice Pilaf

Brown rice pilaf is a nutrient-packed side dish that works nicely with numerous entrees. Brown rice is a whole grain that's rich in fiber, vitamins, and minerals. You may personalize it with your choice of veggies and spices to suit your taste.

These side dishes are meant to complement your main meals with their nutrition and tastes. Whether you like the simplicity of steamed broccoli with garlic and lemon, the diversity of quinoa and vegetable stir-fry, or the vivid spinach and strawberry salad, each side dish is meant to be both tasty and supportive of your prostate health.

Chapter 8

Sweet Endings with a Healthy Twist

Guilt-Free Desserts
Ending a dinner with a great dessert doesn't have to be linked with guilt. In this part, we'll examine a selection of guilt-free dessert choices meant to please your sweet taste while keeping your prostate health in mind.

1. Berry Parfait

A berry parfait is a guilt-free treat that combines Greek yogurt with fresh berries and a drizzle of honey. Greek yogurt delivers protein and probiotics, while berries are rich in antioxidants. The natural sweetness of honey binds it all together, providing a delightful and prostate-friendly treat.

2. Chocolate Avocado Mousse

Chocolate avocado mousse is a rich and decadent dessert that substitutes heavy cream with the healthful fats of avocados. It's sweetened with dark chocolate and a hint of honey, delivering a delightful and guilt-free choice for chocolate lovers.

3. Baked Apples with Cinnamon

Baked apples with cinnamon are a warm and soothing dish that needs no effort. Simply core and slice apples, sprinkle them with cinnamon, and bake until they're soft. This dessert is low in added sugars and rich in fiber, making it a healthy solution for those sweet cravings.

4. Chia Seed Pudding

Chia seed pudding is a flexible and nutrient-rich dish. Chia seeds absorb moisture and become gel-like, providing a pudding-like texture. You may sweeten it with a touch of honey or maple syrup and top it with fresh fruits for extra taste and benefits.

5. Frozen Banana Pops

Frozen banana pops are a fun and kid-friendly snack that can also be enjoyed by adults. Simply skewer banana slices, dip them in dark chocolate, then roll them in chopped almonds or shredded coconut. Freeze until the chocolate is set for a delightful and healthy dessert choice.

6. Yogurt and Fruit Sundaes

Yogurt and fruit sundaes are a simple and adaptable treat. Layer Greek yogurt with fresh fruit like berries, mango, or kiwi, then top it with a sprinkling of granola for additional crunch. This dessert contains delicious protein, vitamins, and fiber deliciously.

7. Fruit Salad with Mint

A fruit salad with mint is a delicious and low-calorie dessert that blends a range of fresh fruits with the fragrant touch of mint leaves. Mint not only offers a burst of flavor but also assists in digestion, making this dessert both tasty and helpful for your general well-being.

8. Oatmeal Raisin Cookies

Oatmeal raisin cookies may be made healthy by using whole wheat flour, and oats, and lowering the sugar amount. You may sweeten them with natural alternatives like honey or maple syrup. These cookies include fiber and entire grains, making them a guilt-free treat.

9. Frozen Yogurt Popsicles

Frozen yogurt popsicles are a delightful and refreshing snack that you can cook using Greek yogurt, fresh fruit, and a touch of honey. These popsicles are a terrific alternative to ice cream, giving protein and probiotics while still fulfilling your sweet desires.

10. Coconut Rice Pudding

Coconut rice pudding is a creamy and tropical dish that utilizes coconut milk and whole-grain rice. You may sweeten it with a small quantity of sugar or natural sweeteners. The addition of toasted coconut flakes lends more taste and texture to this delectable delicacy.

11. Almond and Berry Smoothie

An almond and berry smoothie is a clean and nutritious dessert choice. Blend almond milk, mixed berries, a handful of spinach for extra nutrients, and a dash of honey for sweetness. This dessert is rich in vitamins and antioxidants, making it a delightful and guilt-free alternative.

12. Peach and Almond Crumble

A peach and almond crumble is a soothing and fruit-filled dish. It's created with fresh or canned peaches and topped with a crumbly topping that contains whole wheat flour, oats, and sliced almonds. The crumble is mildly sweetened, delivering a warm and prostate-friendly choice.

13. Blueberry Banana Ice Cream

Blueberry banana ice cream is a simple and healthful dish that blends frozen bananas with blueberries. You may combine them into a delicious and dairy-free ice cream. Blueberries are rich in antioxidants and vitamins, while bananas give natural sweetness without additional sweets.

14. Walnut-Date Bars

Walnut-date bars are a nutrient-dense treat that blends the natural sweetness of dates with the crunch of walnuts. Dates are a fantastic source of fiber and critical minerals, while walnuts are rich in healthy fats and protein.

15. Cherry Almond Bites

Cherry almond bites are a bite-sized dessert that blends dried cherries with almond butter. Dried cherries give antioxidants, while almond butter delivers protein and healthy fats. These tiny joys are both handy and beneficial for prostate health.

16. Mango Sorbet

Mango sorbet is a delightful and sweet delicacy prepared with pureed mango and a dash of lime juice. Mangoes are filled with vitamins and antioxidants, making this dish both tasty and excellent for your prostate.

17. Pumpkin Chia Pudding

Pumpkin chia pudding is a seasonal and fiber-rich treat. It blends pumpkin puree with chia seeds and a mixture of warming spices like cinnamon and nutmeg. Pumpkin is a source of vitamins, while chia seeds supply omega-3 fatty acids and protein.

18. Apricot Bliss Balls

Apricot happiness balls are a pleasant and invigorating dessert that blends dried apricots with nuts like almonds. Apricots are rich in vitamins, while almonds give healthful fats and protein. These bite-sized nibbles are both tasty and beneficial for prostate health.

These prostate-healthy sweet snacks provide a range of alternatives to fulfill your sweet desires while emphasizing your prostate health. Whether you like the simplicity of blueberry banana ice cream, the wholesomeness of walnut-date bars, or the refreshing mango sorbet, each sweet treat is meant to be both tasty and supportive of your general well-being. As you continue exploring additional sweet treat ideas in this chapter, you'll find a broad choice of alternatives to fit your taste and nutritional needs, ensuring that your sweet endings are not only wonderful but also health-conscious.

Chapter 9

Weekly Meal Plans

One-Week and One-Month Sample Meal Plans
Maintaining a prostate-healthy diet is simpler when you have a clear strategy in place. In this part, we present you with example meal plans for both one week and one month, aimed to help you make educated decisions and enjoy a range of tasty and prostate-friendly meals.

One-Week Sample Meal Plan

Day 1: Breakfast
- Scrambled eggs with spinach and tomatoes
- Whole grain toast
- Fresh berries

Lunch
- Quinoa and veggie stir-fry
- Mixed green salad with balsamic vinaigrette

Dinner
- Baked salmon with asparagus
- Brown rice
- Steamed broccoli

Snack
- Greek yogurt with honey and almonds

Day 2: Breakfast
- Oatmeal with sliced bananas and walnuts
- A glass of orange juice

Lunch
- Chickpea and vegetable curry
- Whole wheat couscous
- Mixed fruit salad

Dinner
- Grilled chicken breast with a side of roasted Brussels sprouts
- Quinoa salad with mixed veggies

Snack
- Carrot and hummus sticks

Day 3: Breakfast
- Chia seed pudding with mixed fruit
- A piece of whole-grain bread with almond butter

Lunch
- Lentil soup
- Spinach and strawberry salad with a mild vinaigrette

Dinner
- Eggplant Parmesan
- Mixed green salad with lemon-tahini dressing

Snack
1 Sliced apple with cottage cheese

Day 4: Breakfast
- Green smoothie (spinach, banana, almond milk)
- A handful of mixed nuts

Lunch
- Tuna salad with mixed greens
- Whole grain crackers

Dinner
- Sesame-ginger tofu stir-fry
- Brown rice

Snack
- Frozen banana pops

Day 5: Breakfast
- Sliced avocado with whole grain crackers
- Fresh strawberries

Lunch
- Greek salad with feta cheese
- Quinoa salad

Dinner
- Baked chicken with sweet potato and green
beans
- Quinoa and veggie stir-fry

Snack
- Frozen yogurt popsicles

Day 6: Breakfast
- Cottage cheese with pineapple
- A piece of whole-grain toast

Lunch
- Mixed bean salad with a lemon-tahini
dressing
- Carrot and hummus sticks

Dinner
- Grilled portobello mushrooms
- Brown rice pilaf

Snack
- Mixed nuts and dried fruits

Day 7: Breakfast
- Whole grain pancakes with fresh berries and a sprinkle of honey
- A glass of almond milk

Lunch
- Salmon and asparagus foil pack
- Quinoa salad

Dinner
- Chickpea and vegetable curry
- Mixed green salad with balsamic vinaigrette

Snack
- Chia pudding with fresh fruits

One-Month Sample Meal Plan

Week 2

Day 8: Breakfast
- Omelette with mushrooms and spinach
- Whole grain toast
- Mixed berries

Lunch
- Quinoa and veggie stir-fry
- Mixed green salad with lemon-tahini dressing

Dinner
- Baked trout with roasted sweet potatoes
- Steamed asparagus

Snack
- Greek yogurt with honey and almonds

Day 9: Breakfast
- Green smoothie (kale, banana, almond milk)

- A handful of mixed nuts

Lunch
- Lentil and vegetable soup
- Spinach and strawberry salad with balsamic vinaigrette

Dinner
- Grilled chicken breast with quinoa salad
- Mixed fruit salad

Snack
- Sliced apple with almond butter

Day 10: Breakfast
- Chia seed pudding with mixed fruit
- A piece of whole-grain bread with cottage cheese

Lunch
- Mixed bean salad with lemon-tahini dressing
- Carrot and celery sticks with hummus

Dinner
- Seared shrimp with broccoli and brown rice
- Roasted Brussels sprouts

Snack
- Frozen banana pops

Day 11: Breakfast
- Whole grain waffles with fresh strawberries and Greek yogurt
- A glass of orange juice

Lunch
- Tuna salad with mixed greens
- Whole wheat crackers

Dinner
- Baked cod with a side of quinoa and veggie stir-fry
- Steamed broccoli

Snack
- Sliced cucumber with tzatziki

Day 12: Breakfast
- Cottage cheese with pineapple
- A piece of whole-grain toast

Lunch
- Greek salad with feta cheese
- Whole grain couscous

Dinner
- Grilled salmon with asparagus
- Brown rice pilaf

Snack
- Mixed nuts and dried fruits

Day 13: Breakfast
- Sliced avocado with whole grain crackers
- Fresh blueberries

Lunch
- Chickpea and vegetable curry
- Mixed green salad with balsamic vinaigrette

Dinner
- Teriyaki chicken with quinoa salad
- Mixed fruit salad

Snack
- Chocolate avocado mousse

Day 14: Breakfast
- Scrambled eggs with tomatoes and bell peppers
- Whole grain toast
- Mixed berries

Lunch
- Mixed bean salad with a lemon-tahini dressing
- Carrot and hummus sticks

Dinner
- Grilled portobello mushrooms
- Quinoa and veggie stir-fry

Snack
- Frozen yogurt popsicles

Week 3

Day 15: Breakfast
- Oatmeal with sliced bananas and walnuts
- A glass of almond milk

Lunch
- Quinoa and veggie stir-fry
- Mixed green salad with lemon-tahini dressing

Dinner
- Baked trout with sweet potatoes and steamed asparagus

Snack
- Greek yogurt with honey and almonds

Day 16: Breakfast
- Green smoothie (spinach, banana, almond milk)

- A handful of mixed nuts

Lunch
- Lentil and vegetable soup
- Spinach and strawberry salad with balsamic vinaigrette

Dinner
- Grilled chicken breast with quinoa salad
- Mixed fruit salad

Snack
- Sliced apple with almond butter

Day 17: Breakfast
- Chia seed pudding with mixed fruit
- A piece of whole-grain bread with cottage cheese

Lunch
- Mixed bean salad with lemon-tahini dressing
- Carrot and celery sticks with hummus

Dinner
- Seared shrimp with broccoli and brown rice
- Roasted Brussels sprouts

Snack
- Frozen banana pops

Day 18: Breakfast
- Whole grain waffles with fresh strawberries and Greek yogurt
- A glass of orange juice

Lunch
- Tuna salad with mixed greens
- Whole wheat crackers

Dinner
- Baked cod with quinoa and veggie stir-fry
- Steamed broccoli

Snack
- Sliced cucumber with tzatziki

Day 19: Breakfast
- Cottage cheese with pineapple
- A piece of whole-grain toast

Lunch
- Greek salad with feta cheese
- Whole grain couscous

Dinner
- Grilled salmon with asparagus
- Brown rice pilaf

Snack
- Mixed nuts and dried fruits

Day 20: Breakfast
- Sliced avocado with whole grain crackers
- Fresh blueberries

Lunch
- Chickpea and vegetable curry
- Mixed green salad with balsamic vinaigrette

Dinner
- Teriyaki chicken with quinoa salad
- Mixed fruit salad

Snack
- Chocolate avocado mousse

Day 21: Breakfast
- Scrambled eggs with tomatoes and bell peppers
- Whole grain toast
- Mixed berries

Lunch
- Mixed bean salad with a lemon-tahini dressing
- Carrot and hummus sticks

Dinner
- Grilled portobello mushrooms
- Quinoa and veggie stir-fry

Snack
- Frozen yogurt popsicles

Week 4

Day 22: Breakfast
- Oatmeal with sliced bananas and walnuts
- A glass of almond milk

Lunch
- Quinoa and veggie stir-fry
- Mixed green salad with lemon-tahini dressing

Dinner
- Baked trout with sweet potatoes and steamed asparagus

Snack
- Greek yogurt with honey and almonds

Day 23: Breakfast
- Green smoothie (spinach, banana, almond milk)
- A handful of mixed nuts

Lunch
- Lentil and vegetable soup
- Spinach and strawberry salad with balsamic vinaigrette

Dinner
- Grilled chicken breast with quinoa salad
- Mixed fruit salad

Snack
- Sliced apple with almond butter

Day 24: Breakfast
- Chia seed pudding with mixed fruit
- A piece of whole-grain bread with cottage cheese

Lunch
- Mixed bean salad with lemon-tahini dressing
- Carrot and celery sticks with hummus

Dinner
- Seared shrimp with broccoli and brown rice
- Roasted Brussels sprouts

Snack
- Frozen banana pops

Day 25: Breakfast
- Whole grain waffles with fresh strawberries and Greek yogurt
- A glass of orange juice

Lunch
- Tuna salad with mixed greens
- Whole wheat crackers

Dinner
- Baked cod with quinoa and veggie stir-fry
- Steamed broccoli

Snack
- Sliced cucumber with tzatziki

Day 26: Breakfast
- Cottage cheese with pineapple
- A piece of whole-grain toast

Lunch
- Greek salad with feta cheese
- Whole grain couscous

Dinner
- Grilled salmon with asparagus
- Brown rice pilaf

Snack
- Mixed nuts and dried fruits

Day 27: Breakfast
- Sliced avocado with whole grain crackers
- Fresh blueberries

Lunch
- Chickpea and vegetable curry
- Mixed green salad with balsamic vinaigrette

Dinner
- Teriyaki chicken with quinoa salad
- Mixed fruit salad

Snack
- Chocolate avocado mousse

Day 28: Breakfast
- Scrambled eggs with tomatoes and bell peppers
- Whole grain toast
- Mixed berries

Lunch
- Mixed bean salad with a lemon-tahini dressing
- Carrot and hummus sticks

Dinner
- Grilled portobello mushrooms
- Quinoa and veggie stir-fry

Snack
- Frozen yogurt popsicles

Week 5

Day 29: Breakfast
- Oatmeal with sliced bananas and walnuts
- A glass of almond milk

Lunch
- Quinoa and veggie stir-fry
- Mixed green salad with lemon-tahini dressing

Dinner
- Baked trout with sweet potatoes and steamed asparagus

Snack
- Greek yogurt with honey and almonds

Day 30: Breakfast
- Green smoothie (spinach, banana, almond milk)
- A handful of mixed nuts

Lunch
- Lentil and vegetable soup
- Spinach and strawberry salad with balsamic vinaigrette

Dinner
- Grilled chicken breast with quinoa salad
- Mixed fruit salad

Snack
- Sliced apple with almond butter

Day 31: Breakfast
- Chia seed pudding with mixed fruit
- A piece of whole-grain bread with cottage cheese

Lunch
- Mixed bean salad with lemon-tahini dressing
- Carrot and celery sticks with hummus

Dinner
- Seared shrimp with broccoli and brown rice
- Roasted Brussels sprouts

Snack
- Frozen banana pops

Throughout this last week of the one-month sample meal plan, you've continued to enjoy a varied assortment of tasty and prostate-healthy foods. These strategies are meant to help you make educated decisions and enjoy a range of enjoyable alternatives as you try to preserve prostate health. Feel free to adapt the programs depending on your tastes and nutritional requirements, and continue on your road toward greater health.

Grocery Lists for Easy Planning

To make your prostate-healthy meal planning as simple as possible, we've developed complete shopping lists to help you keep organized and efficient. These lists are grouped to ease your buying experience:

Protein:
- Salmon
- Tuna
- Chicken breast
- Shrimp
- Tofu
- Eggs

Fruits:
- Berries (blueberries, strawberries, raspberries)
- Bananas
- Apples
- Oranges
- Kiwi
- Avocado
- Pineapple
- Fresh berries (strawberries, blueberries)
- Fresh fruits (apples, oranges, etc.)

Vegetables:
- Spinach
- Kale
- Broccoli
- Asparagus
- Bell peppers
- Tomatoes
- Eggplant
- Brussels sprouts
- Green beans
- Sweet potatoes
- Carrots
- Celery
- Cucumber
- Zucchini
- Mushrooms
- Mixed greens (lettuce, arugula, etc.)
- Mixed veggies (for stir-fries)
- Fresh herbs (parsley, cilantro, mint, etc.)

Grains:
- Quinoa
- Brown rice
- Whole grain pasta

- Whole wheat bread
- Whole wheat crackers
- Oats
- Whole grain waffles
- Whole wheat couscous

Legumes:
- Chickpeas
- Lentils
- Mixed beans

Dairy and Alternatives:
- Greek yogurt
- Almond milk
- Cottage cheese

Nuts and Seeds:
- Walnuts
- Almonds
- Chia seeds

Oils and Condiments:
- Olive oil
- Balsamic vinaigrette

- Lemon-tahini dressing
- Tzatziki
- Teriyaki sauce

Herbs and Spices:
- Garlic
- Ginger
- Cinnamon
- Nutmeg
- Paprika
- Sesame seeds

Miscellaneous:
- Honey
- Dark chocolate (for chocolate mousse)
- Cocoa powder (for chocolate mousse)
- Dried fruits (for snacking)
- Hummus
- Whole wheat crackers

These classified grocery lists give a straightforward and quick method to organize your shopping visits and ensure you have all the required supplies available to create your prostate-healthy meals. Feel free to alter these lists depending on your tastes and dietary requirements, and continue enjoying delectable, nutritious, and supporting meals for your prostate health.

Chapter 10

Lifestyle Tips for Prostate Health

Exercise and Physical Activity
Maintaining a healthy lifestyle is vital for prostate health. In this part, we'll investigate the role of exercise and physical activity in fostering a healthy prostate.

The Impact of Exercise on Prostate Health
Regular exercise gives several advantages for general well-being, including the health of the prostate. Here's how exercise may favorably benefit your prostate:

- Reduced Risk of Prostate Cancer: Studies have revealed that men who participate in regular physical exercise are less likely to get prostate cancer.

Exercise helps control hormones and decrease inflammation, variables linked with a reduced risk of prostate cancer.

- Improved Prostate Function: Physical exercise improves prostate function. Regular exercise may help ease symptoms of benign prostatic hyperplasia (BPH), a non-cancerous enlargement of the prostate that can lead to urinary difficulties.

- Weight Management: Maintaining a healthy weight via exercise is vital. Obesity is associated with a greater risk of prostate cancer, and regular physical exercise may help control weight and minimize this risk.

- Enhanced Immune Function: Exercise improves the immune system, which is crucial for general health and may play a role in defending against numerous illnesses, including prostate cancer.

- Cardiovascular Health: Prostate health is intimately connected to cardiovascular health. Physical exercise may lessen the risk of heart disease and, in turn, contribute to improved prostate health.

Exercise Recommendations for Prostate Health

To obtain the advantages of exercise for prostate health, consider the following recommendations:

- Aim for Regular Activity: Engage in at least 150 minutes of moderate-intensity aerobic exercise or 75 minutes of vigorous-intensity aerobic activity every week. This might be brisk walking, cycling, swimming, or other activities that get your heart rate up.

- Strength Training: Incorporate strength training workouts at least two days a week. These workouts, utilizing weights or resistance bands, assist in preserving muscular mass and bone density.

- Flexibility and Balance: Include flexibility and balance workouts in your program. Yoga or Pilates may increase flexibility and lessen the chance of injury.

- Consult a Healthcare Professional: Before beginning a new workout regimen, particularly if you have current health issues, visit your healthcare professional. They can give counsel targeted to your requirements.

- Stay Hydrated: Proper hydration is vital during activity. Dehydration may lead to health concerns, so drink lots of water before, during, and after your activity.

- Listen to Your Body: Pay heed to your body's messages. If you encounter pain, dizziness, or other discomfort while activity, stop and seek medical help if required.

Regular physical exercise is a cornerstone of a healthy lifestyle that promotes prostate health. By including exercise in your daily routine, you may minimize your risk of prostate difficulties, control your weight, and enhance your general well-being.

Stress Management and Mindful Eating

The Impact of Stress on Prostate Health

Stress is a part of life, but persistent stress may have a bad influence on your general health, including your prostate. High-stress levels may lead to different health difficulties, and there is evidence showing a relationship between chronic stress and prostate cancer.

Chronic stress may lead to:

- Inflammation: Long-term stress may promote inflammation in the body, which is a risk factor for prostate cancer.

- Unhealthy Behaviors: Many individuals resort to unhealthy coping techniques when stressed, such as overeating, smoking, or excessive alcohol use, which may have a bad influence on prostate health.

- Hormonal Changes: Stress may lead to hormonal changes that may harm the prostate.

Stress Management Strategies for Prostate Health

Effective stress management may lead to greater prostate health. Here are some techniques to help you handle stress:

1. Exercise: As noted before, regular physical exercise is a good stress reducer. It releases endorphins, which are natural mood lifters.

2. Mindfulness and Meditation: Practicing mindfulness and meditation may help decrease stress and promote mental well-being.

3. Deep Breathing: Deep, steady breaths help soothe your nervous system and lessen tension.

4. Support Systems: Share your worries with friends, family, or a therapist. Talking about your stresses might be beneficial.

5. Time Management: Efficiently managing your time and creating realistic objectives helps lessen stress connected to work or duties.

Mindful Eating for Prostate Health

Mindful eating is a discipline that encourages you to pay attention to the sensation of eating and your body's hunger and fullness indicators. It may be useful for prostate health in numerous ways:

1. Portion Control: Mindful eating helps you identify when you've had enough to eat, reducing overeating and promoting a healthy weight.

2. Balanced Nutrition: Being conscious of what you eat may support balanced and healthy dietary choices, which are vital for prostate health.

3. Digestive Health: Eating slowly and thoughtfully may improve digestion, minimizing pain and bloating.

4. Emotional Eating: It may assist in uncovering emotional triggers for poor eating patterns and suggest better strategies to deal with stress.

Mindful Eating Tips:

- Eat without distractions: Turn off the TV and put away your phone during mealtime.

- Savor each bite: Pay attention to the flavor, texture, and scent of your meal.

- Listen to your body: Eat when you're hungry and quit when you're full.

- Avoid rushing: Take your time to savor your food.

- remain hydrated: Drink water to remain hydrated, since dehydration may often be misconstrued with hunger.

By controlling stress and practicing mindful eating, you may enhance your overall well-being and promote your prostate health. In the following part, we'll discuss the value of frequent check-ups and early detection in preserving your prostate health.

Hydration and Staying Healthy

Hydration for Prostate Health
Adequate hydration is crucial to sustaining your prostate health and general well-being. Here's how being adequately hydrated may benefit your prostate:

1. Urinary Health: Staying hydrated helps avoid urinary tract infections and minimizes the likelihood of disorders associated with the prostate, such as benign prostatic hyperplasia (BPH).

2. Digestive Health: Proper water helps good digestion, lowering the chance of constipation and other gastrointestinal issues.

3. Nutrient Absorption: Water is crucial for the absorption of key nutrients, particularly those that promote prostate health.

How to Stay Hydrated:

- Drink lots of water throughout the day. Aim for at least 8-10 glasses (approximately 2-2.5 liters) per day, although individual requirements may vary.

- Consume hydrating meals like fruits and vegetables, which have high water content.

- Limit dehydrating drinks like coffee and alcohol.

- Listen to your body's cues; thirst is an indication that your body needs more water.

Staying Healthy for Prostate Health

A proactive attitude to remaining healthy may dramatically lower the chance of prostate troubles. Here are some essential tips:

1. Regular Check-ups: Schedule frequent check-ups with your healthcare practitioner, including prostate-specific tests, particularly as you age. Early identification may be key for controlling and treating prostate disorders efficiently.

2. Smoking Cessation: If you smoke, consider stopping. Smoking is related to an

increased risk of prostate cancer and other health risks.

3. Limit Alcohol Consumption: Excessive alcohol consumption might lead to prostate issues. If you want to drink, do so in moderation.

4. Safe Sun Exposure: Adequate vitamin D is crucial for prostate health. Spend time in the sun to increase natural vitamin D production but protect your skin from excessive UV exposure.

5. Sleep: Prioritize quality sleep. Sleep is vital for general health, including prostate health.

6. Regular Physical Activity: Maintain your exercise program for general well-being and prostate health.

7. Emotional Health: Manage stress with relaxation methods, hobbies, or obtaining help from a therapist.

8. Proactive Health Monitoring: Be mindful of any signs that may signal prostate concerns, such as changes in urine patterns or pain, and quickly visit a healthcare expert.

9. Healthy Relationships: Maintaining strong connections with family and friends may give emotional support, decreasing stress and increasing well-being.

By following these hydration and general health suggestions, you may maintain your prostate health and lower the risk of prostate-related illnesses. Staying proactive and adopting mindful lifestyle choices may lead to a healthier and more meaningful life.

Chapter 11

Personal Testimonials from Prostate Health Journey

In this chapter, we'll present the genuine experiences of people who have launched their paths toward improved prostate health. These personal testimonies illustrate the difficulties, victories, and significant insights learned from their experiences. It is our aim that these tales may inspire and drive you on your road to prostate health.

John's Journey: Finding Strength in Exercise

John, a 58-year-old retired teacher, was diagnosed with prostate cancer in his early

50s. Initially, the news seemed overwhelming, but he vowed to adopt a proactive attitude. John started exercising frequently, a routine that provided him not just physical strength but mental resilience.

"I began by taking daily walks. Gradually, I moved up to jogging, and then I joined a local exercise class. The support of the group, the fresh air, and the physical exertion did wonders for my spirit. It helped me deal with the stress of diagnosis and therapy."

John's tale underscores the necessity of physical exercise in preserving emotional well-being along the prostate health journey.

Lisa's Lessons: Mindful Eating for a Healthier Life

Lisa, a 47-year-old dietician, is always focused on helping people make smart dietary choices. However, her path toward prostate health started when she began investigating dietary advice for her husband, who was diagnosed with an enlarged prostate.

"As I went into the study, I realized that I had ignored my health. I was balancing my job, family, and assisting my spouse, but I wasn't prioritizing myself. Mindful eating proved a game-changer for both of us. We began preparing balanced, healthful meals together, and it drew us closer. It's not only about the food; it's about sustaining our bodies and our connection."

Lisa's experience highlights the transformational impact of mindful eating, not just for physical health but for establishing connections within relationships.

Henry's Healing: A Supportive Network

Henry, a 63-year-old retired engineer, confronted prostate cancer with tenacity and the support of friends and family.

"My diagnosis was a shock, but I was lucky to have a wonderful support network. My friends and family were there every step of the way. We learned about prostate health together, and their support made all the difference. It's crucial to have friends that care about you and help you remain optimistic."

Henry's story underlines the need for emotional support and having a network of individuals who are there for you throughout your prostate health journey.

These personal testimonies remind us that each journey is unique, and there is no one-size-fits-all approach to prostate health. The tales of John, Lisa, and Henry indicate that by embracing exercise, mindful nutrition, and creating a strong support network, you can overcome hurdles and achieve success on your way to improved prostate health. In the following sections, we will give extra materials and information to help your journey.

Conclusion

Taking Control of Your Prostate Health

Your prostate health journey is a significant element of your overall well-being. In the course of this book, we've addressed the necessity of understanding prostate cancer, the influence of food and nutrition, and the role of lifestyle choices in maintaining your prostate health. We've heard personal testimonies and learned from real-life events that give inspiration and vital insights.

Taking Control of Your Prostate Health

Prostate health is a journey that demands your active involvement. It's about making educated choices, from food habits to exercise routines, from stress management to developing a support network. By taking charge of your prostate health, you empower yourself to live a better, happier life. Remember these crucial takeaways:

- Regular check-ups are vital for early detection and treatment.
- Maintain a diet rich in prostate-healthy foods, and practice mindful eating.
- Prioritize physical activity and exercise for a healthy prostate and general well-being.
- Manage stress properly and nurture your emotional wellness.
- Stay hydrated to assist your prostate and your body as a whole.
- Proactive health monitoring may make a major impact on your path.
- Don't hesitate to seek assistance and direction from healthcare experts, friends, and family.

Resources for Further Reading and Support

Your road to prostate health extends beyond the pages of this book. There are innumerable tools available to assist you to get greater information, find support, and remain inspired. Here are some avenues to explore:

- Healthcare Providers: Your main healthcare practitioner is your initial point of contact for prostate health. Regular check-ups and open communication are crucial.

- Support Groups: Local and online support groups link you with people who are on similar paths. Sharing experiences and expertise may be incredibly useful.

- Books: Numerous publications dive into prostate health, giving in-depth information on different facets of the issue.

- Websites: Reputable websites, such as those from cancer groups, provide excellent information and tools on prostate health.

- Nutrition and Health Experts: Consult licensed dietitians, nutritionists, or other healthcare specialists for specialized counsel.

- Fitness Professionals: Personal trainers and fitness specialists can help you build training regimens specific to your requirements.

- Mental Health Professionals: Therapists and counselors may help your emotional well-being and stress management.

- Community Health Programs: Local community centers regularly hold workshops and events relevant to prostate health and wellbeing.

Remember that your journey is unique, and the route to prostate health is a very personalized one. Seek out the tools and help that connect with you and fit with your personal needs and objectives.

In conclusion, we urge you to continue learning, developing, and aiming for improved prostate health. With the information and insights obtained from this book and the support of healthcare experts, friends, and family, you are well-equipped to take charge of your prostate health and have a full life. Your health is your most significant possession, and your road toward prostate health is a journey toward a happier and healthier future.

Dear Readers,

I hope this communication finds you well. I am writing to offer my thanks for your assistance in perusing the pages of "Prostate cancer diet cookbook for beginners." Your path toward improved prostate health is vital, and I genuinely hope the book has been a beneficial resource for you.

If you've found the material enlightening, or if the book has had a significant influence on your knowledge of prostate health, I would appreciate it if you could take a minute to share your comments with others. Your honest evaluations may help other readers make educated judgments about the book.

Whether on online merchants, social media, or book review venues, your input is incredibly useful. Your reviews add not just to the book's exposure but also to the community's cumulative knowledge of prostate health.

Thank you for being a part of this adventure, and I look forward to hearing your opinions on "prostate cancer diet cookbook for beginners." Your support means the world to me.

Warm regards,

Kimberly Talbot